The ADD Myth

The ADD Myth

How to Cultivate the Unique Gifts of Intense Personalities

MARTHA BURGE

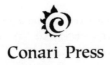

Conari Press

First published in 2012 by Conari Press
Red Wheel/Weiser, LLC
With offices at:
665 Third Street, Suite 400
San Francisco, CA 94107
www.redwheelweiser.com

ISBN: 978-1-57324-582-1

Library of Congress Cataloging-in-Publication Data
Burge, Martha.
   The ADD myth : how to cultivate the unique gifts of intense personalities /
   Martha Burge.
      p. cm.
   ISBN 978-1-57324-582-1
1. Attention-deficit hyperactivity disorder. 2. Behavior disorders in children. I. Title.
II. Title: Attention deficit disorder myth.
   RJ506.H9B87 2012
   618.92'8589—dc23   2012010793

Cover by Jim Warner
Cover art by Christopher Oates/Shutterstock.com
Interior by Dutton & Sherman

10 9 8 7 6 5 4 3 2 1

Printed in the United States of America
MAL

The paper used in this publication meets the minimum requirements of the American National Standard for Information Sciences—Permanence of Paper for Printed Library Materials Z39.48-1992 (R1997).

This book is dedicated to my sons, Stephan and Adam, who have taught me a depth of love I never imagined. Raising them has been the greatest joy of my life. They showed me the beautiful spirit in intensity and inspired my life's work.

CONTENTS

FOREWORD

Martha Burge's book is a useful response to the recent "epidemic" of attention deficit disorder. When we published DSM-IV in 1994, the rate in children was just a bit more than 3 percent. Now, it has almost tripled to a remarkable 10 percent. The diagnosis of ADD has also exploded in adults, with rates jumping from under 2 percent to as much as 5 percent. And this diagnostic inflation is not just a local United States phenomenon; it is happening simultaneously in all the developed countries around the world.

Ms. Burge offers a strategy she hopes may help cure the "epidemic" of ADD. She warns us to stop medicalizing what is often basically normal behavior and to stop over-treating with unnecessary and potentially harmful medication. She offers an alternative approach for dealing with the "myth" of ADD that accepts and accommodates the human variability it represents, rather than pathologizing and treating as illness all hyperactivity, impulsivity, and distractability.

Let's first explore the causes of the ADD "epidemic"—this will help us understand how best to contain it. A small part of the growth in ADD rates was a predictable result of changes we made in its DSM-IV definition. Previous definitions required hyperactivity, impulsivity, and inattentiveness. We recognized that some people with ADD (particularly females) have clinically significant inattentiveness, but without the hyperactivity or impulsivity. Our field testing predicted that allowing for this in our DSM-IV definition would increase rates of ADD by about 15 percent.

But none of us working on DSM-IV imagined there would be a tripling of rates in so short a period of time. We weren't psychic and had no way of predicting the other two events that soon completely changed the ADD landscape. Shortly after DSM-IV was published, new and expensive on-patent ADHD drugs were approved for marketing by the Food and Drug Administration. The previous generic drugs were so cheap and unprofitable that drug companies didn't bother to push their sales. Now, with potential blockbusters in hand, they had powerful financial incentives to aggressively extend their market by promoting the diagnosis of ADD and encouraging its medication treatment.

And, almost simultaneously (for unrelated reasons), the FDA deregulated some of its control over drug company marketing. It gave Big Pharma permission to advertise its pills not only to doctors but also directly to consumers. Soon, the companies were mounting expensive and ubiquitous promotional campaigns in print media and on TV and the Internet. Total marketing budgets grew from an already hefty $791 million in 1999 to an astounding $4.8 billion in 2006. A small but significant fraction of this consisted of a highly successful marketing campaign to convince psychiatrists, pediatricians, family practitioners, parents, patients, and teachers that ADD was under-recognized and under-treated. ADD became a fashionable fad diagnosis and drug sales took off—from $304 million in 1994; to $658 million in 1999; to $2.11 billion by 2003.

Ms. Burge correctly worries that the drug companies have succeeded in their campaign to re-label as mental disorder what is often just a normal variation in behavior. As a consequence, the use of ADD drugs has doubled, so that almost 5 percent of our children are now receiving a pill for it (with an even higher percentage among boys). Loose diagnosis and careless prescription bring questionable benefit but accrue considerable costs and risks. Although medication clearly helps in the short term, its long-term benefits are unclear. Often there are side effects (like insomnia and decreased appetite), and the long-term risks (especially for kids with their developing brains) are unknown. Inaccurate diagnosis may unleash stigma and cause a reduced sense of self-control. And then there is the serious problem of the secondary market for diverted stimulant drugs. Illegal stimulant use for recreation and performance enhancement already occurs in up to 10 percent of high schoolers and up to 35 percent of college students.

DSM-5, a new revision of the diagnostic system, is scheduled to appear in May, 2013. Unfortunately, it will markedly increase the current diagnostic inflation and open the floodgates to even greater overmedication. The DSM-5 redefinition of ADD further reduces diagnostic thresholds and makes it even easier for kids, and especially for adults, to be misdiagnosed and over-treated. I see absolutely no justification for this further expansion of an already bloated diagnosis. Unless there is a huge public outcry or government intervention, DSM-5 will blow up the ADD bubble even further.

Many people make the false assumption that the experts working on DSM-5 must be expanding the diagnosis of ADD because they are in bed with the drug companies and want to help them sell pills by expanding the market of potential customers. I strongly disagree. The DSM-5 experts have an intellectual, but not a financial, conflict of interest. They are making very bad decisions, but for pure motives. Experts tend to overvalue their pet diagnosis, worry about missed cases, underestimate the risks of over-diagnosis, and ignore that ADD is often diagnosed carelessly—especially in primary care settings by rushed practitioners who are much less expert than they. DSM-5 will be a great boon to drug company sales and profits—but that will be a side effect of DSM-5, not its intent.

Martha Burge cures the worrisome ADD "epidemic" by turning ADD instead into a "myth." She correctly points out that symptoms of hyperactivity, impulsivity, and inattention are very common in the general population—really no more than part of the Bell curve distribution of individual difference. ADD is not a clearly defined illness diagnosable with an objective, biological test. There is no bright line delineating where to draw the boundary between normality and disorder. Burge considers ADD to be a harmful myth that errs by seeing the glass half empty. She presents a contrasting half-full perspective that celebrates the emotional intensity and breadth of attention that is currently mislabeled ADD: "With a greater range of attention we are never inattentive; we are always taking in more than others."

Burge decries the ADD "myth" as a medicalization of emotional intensity. She would prefer we accommodate human difference, rather than explain it away as an ill to be casually treated with a pill. Burge normalizes what the DSM pathologizes. She recommends that we not be preoccupied with the limitations and impairments that come with ADD. Instead, Burge focuses on the benefits inherent in an ADD lifestyle, and suggests ways to enhance them further and to limit and cope with the concomitant difficulties.

Readers will feel engaged, understood, and inspired and will find a wealth of practical tips and useful information. Ms. Burge uses her experience and wisdom to turn what may have seemed like problems into opportunities for growth and discovery. Her style is lively, accessible, vivid, and intimate. For many people diagnosed with mild or nonexistent ADD, her techniques may be an effective way to a better life and may reduce or eliminate the need for medication.

I agree with much of Burge's approach and think it is a useful deterrent to diagnostic inflation and pill pushing. But she and I do have a definite parting of the ways. Burge describes ADD as harmful "myth." I see it more as an overdone fad. We both agree that ADD is currently being wildly overdiagnosed, but Burge would get rid of it altogether, while I endorse ADD as a useful diagnosis when cautiously and correctly applied to the small percentage of people at the far extreme of the Bell curve in their hyperactivity, impulsivity, and inattention. ADD should be diagnosed when the problems have started in early childhood; are severe, persistent, and classic in presentation; and cause unremitting and unacceptable impairment at school and at home. In these extreme cases, a diagnosis of ADD makes sense, and—when nothing else has worked—medication is often useful, and sometimes absolutely necessary.

So, I agree with Burge that a good deal of the current ADD hoopla is "myth," and I applaud her methods for dispelling it. But I think she goes too far in altogether denying the existence of ADD and in dismissing the sometimes essential role of medication. This is the perfect book for the many with mild or nonexistent ("mythic") ADD, but it may be misleading for the few with severe and classic ADD that has not been managed sufficiently without medication. Everyone should try the techniques taught by Ms. Burge, but we shouldn't expect they will always be enough by themselves to get the job done. And people shouldn't feel like failures if they don't work. Medicine should not be a casually overused first line intervention, but it is nice to have in reserve when other interventions like the ones suggested here are not enough.

Allen Frances, MD
Chair, DSM-IV Task Force
Professor Emeritus and former Chair
Department of Psychiatry
Duke University

A NOTE TO READERS

Other people may have told you there's something wrong with you. They may have said you are damaged and labeled you disordered. But what if that is not true? This book reveals the underlying condition responsible for many misdiagnoses of mental disorder, particularly ADD. It explains both the symptoms that often result in a diagnosis and the reasons for the complexity of your character. It's not too late for you.

INTRODUCTION

This is a place where you are welcomed,
where people big and small who save insects from the pool are
*   cherished,*
where your next big idea is taken seriously and supported with
*   a whole heart,*
and where the curiosity that leads you to obsess on something
*   for hours or days on end is understood and no one will men-*
*   tion the stack of mail on the desk.*
Welcome to a world where dancing, pacing, and chattering are
*   to be expected,*
where it's understood that the next great project is all consum-
*   ing, as it should be,*
where even your quickness to anger is met with understanding
*   of the frustration behind it,*
and the underlying dissatisfaction with all that is wrong in
*   the world, which strikes your moral outrage and sometimes*
*   leaves you feeling powerless, can be set aside for a short*
*   while.*
Here the strength and beauty of your spirit is valued,
deep frustrations that keep you awake at night are soothed,
and you are free to share your naturally sensitive, creative,
*   gifted, and unique soul in a safe place.*

Those that would say that you are too sensitive, too emotional,
  too active, or too different are banned.
Welcome to a place where you can finally relax and be yourself,
  where the weight of matters beyond your control is lifted,
  and you can play again.
You are my people, and I am honored to have you here.

There is a strangeness about certain people that fascinates me. I can recognize it very quickly now by the spark in a person's eye, a certain determined quickness in the gait, or the lovely flowing way a conversation can get carried away and lead down uncharted paths. Whenever I meet this type of person, my heart quickens. They are my people. I didn't have a name for them until my firstborn child was diagnosed with ADHD.

As I started to write about the unique qualities of these people I had come to call "intense," I found that while it sounds a lot like ADHD, it's so much richer. There is a deep sensitivity, a fullness of experience, a capacity for fantasy and creativity, and an intellectual curiosity that seems to define them so much more than the one-sided, negative descriptions found for ADHD do. At that time I had identified intellectual, emotional, and creative intensity. I read everything I could find on the subject of intensity and stumbled upon Dr. Kazimierz Dabrowski. This man had already spent a lifetime on this very same path. He used different terms both for the perceived disorder and the underlying condition, but his perspective was identical to mine. His work has allowed me to progress in my work as if he had personally held out a hand and pulled me up.

I blended his work with my own and others'. When it began to come together into a single cohesive approach, I felt that something special had emerged. As I shared it with my coaching clients, they said it was the missing piece.

The realization that the true condition of those often diagnosed with ADHD is intensity was a bittersweet epiphany. I wish I had known this when my children were young. I wish I'd had a clue about it when I was young. There were so many missed opportunities and so many times when I felt, as you may have felt, too different and in many ways not good enough. Now I'm grateful to be able to share the truth and a path out of disorder with others, and I hope that it may make as profound a difference in their lives. I've found that intensity, when nurtured, is the greatest asset a person can have if they want to achieve really big things, bring about change, or create new and exciting possibilities.

You'll notice that while I use the more commonly recognized term "ADD" (attention deficit disorder) in the title, I use the correct term "ADHD" (attention deficit/hyperactivity disorder) throughout the rest of the book. It's a technicality, but I don't want it to confuse anyone. The term "ADD" was only used by the DSM (*Diagnostic and Statistical Manual of Mental Disorders*) from 1980 to 1987.

This book is organized and clearly labeled so that you can get the information you want when you want it. You have my permission (not that you need it) to read this book in any way that works for you. To that end I include summaries of the main points for the impatient at the end of each chapter. Feel free to hit the high points and move on or dally in the stories and details for a deeper understanding. The practices to develop each of the intensities are designed to culminate in an understanding of how to use your intensities to achieve whatever you want in life.

1

There Is No Such Thing as ADHD

The hardest part about gaining any new idea is sweeping out the false idea occupying that niche. As long as that niche is occupied, evidence and proof and logical demonstration get nowhere. But once the niche is emptied of the wrong idea that has been filling it—once you can honestly say, "I don't know," then it becomes possible to get at the truth.
—ROBERT A. HEINLEIN, THE CAT WHO
WALKS THROUGH WALLS

I know I have very few standing beside me in my stance that there is no such thing as ADHD. The vast majority of psychiatrists, psychologists, educators, parents, and others believe at their core that ADHD is truly a disorder. I'm not anticipating that this little book will change their minds. The ideas they have are well substantiated by years of practice and documentation. The longer these ideas exist, the more valid they appear.

I contend that while perhaps well-meaning, this description of intense people as having a disorder is a farce. Millions of people have been taken in by it, and most of them believe that their participation in the farce is in the best interest of their patients, their children, and

1

themselves. It is with great conviction that I tell you that labeling these people as disordered not only is an error, but also contributes to creating the dis-ease it intends to treat by withholding the understanding and development of their true intense and gifted nature.

THE DSM AND A CULTURE OF DISORDER

ADHD began as a construct in someone's mind. Psychiatrists see mental disorders or potential signs of mental disorder in every patient that presents to them. The very fact that a person goes to see a psychiatrist means that the psychiatrist must find a diagnosis in order to bill for the visit. It's a reward system. Find a diagnosis, get paid. It's that simple. The possible diagnoses are found in the DSM, which is created by consensus of a group of people who regularly get together and publish a book. This book contains descriptions of every mental disorder. By definition, if a condition is in the book, it's a disorder; if it's not in the book, it's normal. You can see how important this one book is to the way we see ourselves in this culture.

The DSM is sometimes treated like the Bible of the psychiatric profession. It states its primary purpose is to provide a guide for clinical practice in diagnosing psychiatric disorders. Because we are forever learning about disorders, the DSM goes through a continual review process, resulting in new versions being published every few years. The DSM-5 is scheduled to be released in May 2013.

As happens with manuals like this one, people who use it tend to anoint it with powers beyond its intent. It is sometimes seen to define the entirety of mental health and disorder. Common sense tells us that there is no way a single reference book can include all the information needed to identify every type of mental disorder that exists within the human population. We can also guess that with such a broad scope, there is at least a possibility that the criteria supplied could be used to indicate disorder within what should be healthy human differences. But the glow around the book continues.

Before the first printing of the DSM, little had been done to categorize mental disorders. Each mental hospital had its own system. The federal government was interested in collecting statistics on mental disorders, but the lack of a unified system to categorize these disorders made the effort impossible. As a result, the American Psychiatric Association (APA) took on the challenge to produce a system that could be used nationwide. The first printing of the DSM was based on input from both mental hospitals and the Department of Veterans Affairs. Considering the sources, there wasn't much emphasis on childhood disorders or development.

In 1966 Dr. Samuel Clements wrote an article on minimal brain dysfunction in which he describes a number of learning or behavioral disabilities found in children with average to above-average intelligence. He identified the effect on motor activity and attention span. The label "minimal brain dysfunction" likely resulted from the fact that he believed the cause of these disabilities to be minor damage to the brain stem. This may have been the first formally accepted description of ADHD, although it has been recognized in one form or another by mental health professionals for at least a century.

By the time DSM-II was printed in 1968, the label had been adjusted to "hyperkinetic reaction of childhood or adolescence" with a one-line description: "This disorder is characterized by overactivity, restlessness, distractibility, and short attention span, especially in young children; the behavior usually diminishes in adolescence." This change reflects the APA's efforts to avoid labeling a disorder according to the cause of the disorder, mostly because they knew they were only guessing at the cause. There was no evidence of differences in brain structure or functioning. By this time, Ritalin was already in use to treat hyperactivity.

MEDICATION GOES IN SEARCH OF PATIENTS

Once there was a description of ADHD as a mental disorder and a pharmaceutical treatment option available, the disorder seemed to go in search of patients. This practice is very different than the treatment of any other type of mental disorder. In the case of paranoia or schizophrenia, the patients bring themselves to the doctor for treatment. ADHD goes in search of patients, much like many newly discovered and much-advertised physical ailments such as restless legs syndrome. "Ask your doctor!" It should be no surprise that the pharmaceutical companies are paying for those ads. But are they also funding ADHD awareness?

Medication for ADHD is a multibillion-dollar industry. It's clear that the pharmaceutical companies have a lot to gain from an increase in diagnosis. It's also becoming clear that they have the resources to influence the outcome.

In 1987 CHADD (Children and Adults with ADHD) was founded to support people with ADHD. According to a transcript from *PBS NewsHour*'s Merrow Report, CHADD was funded by Ciba-Geigy, secretly receiving almost $800,000 between 1991 and 1994.[1] I've been involved with CHADD for years. I still am, and this hit me like a ton of bricks. The CHADD website states:

> CHADD was founded in 1987 by a small group of parents
> of children with AD/HD and two treating psychologists in
> Plantation, Florida (near Miami). These parents came together
> because they felt frustrated and isolated, and there were few
> places to turn for support and information about AD/HD.[2]

However, they also state that pharmaceutical donations received by CHADD as of June 30, 2009, included support from Eli Lilly, McNeil, Novartis, and Shire US. This constitutes 39.5 percent of CHADD's total revenue, or about $1.5 million, in 2009. This fact by itself is not as troublesome as the fact that these arrangements were kept secret for so long.

The use of stimulant medication to treat ADHD in children in the United States has grown from 2.4 percent in 1996 to 3.5 percent in 2008. That's a half million more children on drugs.[3] The drug is introduced to parents as a safe treatment plan. Indeed it's not very hard to find supporting articles and studies showing that taking stimulants under a doctor's supervision for treatment of ADHD is safe. But the very same people will also tell you that stimulants are deadly. The list of potential serious side effects of stimulant use contains paranoia, anxiety, depression, tachycardia (increased heart rate), dizziness, high blood pressure, increased sweating, decrease in appetite, sleeplessness, and more. One side effect usually attributed to consistent abuse or a serious overdose is amphetamine psychosis. This is similar to the symptoms of schizophrenia. Vivid auditory hallucinations and paranoid delusions are caused by the brain's fear center being overstimulated. This couldn't happen when the drug is prescribed by a doctor and administered as directed, right? Wrong! My son was only ten years old when he began to experience auditory hallucinations while taking a prescribed stimulant for treatment of ADHD. There are other stories about children taking medication for ADHD as prescribed and under a doctor's care that have had even more serious side effects, including death.[4]

I'm not one of those antidrug advocates. I believe in better living through chemistry; it's just that this should be done with a solid understanding of the risks. Drugs should be used only when there are no other options. To prescribe such strong psychotropic drugs to children for an illness that cannot be proven seems irresponsible, particularly if the intent of the prescription is only to improve performance in school.

There's no question that the pharmaceutical companies that manufacture the medications used to treat ADHD stand to benefit from an increase in prevalence. The only remaining question is how much misinformation has been distributed and what part drug manufacturers are playing in today's increase in ADHD diagnosis.

WHY SCHOOLS AND PARENTS SEEK DIAGNOSIS

The symptoms in the diagnostic criteria for ADHD fall into three categories of behavior: inattention, hyperactivity, and impulsivity. The chart below shows the symptoms matched with what the implied "normal" behavior should be.

INATTENTION

	Symptom	Normal
(a)	Often fails to give close attention to details or makes careless mistakes in schoolwork, work, or other activities	Pays close attention to details and rarely makes careless mistakes
(b)	Often has difficulty sustaining attention in tasks or play activities	Sustains attention in tasks
(c)	Often does not seem to listen when spoken to directly	Listens when spoken to directly
(d)	Often does not follow through on instructions and fails to finish schoolwork, chores, or duties in the workplace (not due to oppositional behavior or failure to understand instructions)	Follows through on instructions and finishes schoolwork, chores, etc. without reminders
(e)	Often has difficulty organizing tasks and activities	Has no difficulty organizing tasks and activities

	Symptom	Normal
(f)	Often avoids, dislikes, or is reluctant to engage in tasks that require sustained mental effort (such as schoolwork or homework)	Enjoys engaging in tasks that require sustained mental effort
(g)	Often loses things necessary for tasks or activities (e.g., toys, school assignments, pencils, books, or tools)	Rarely loses things
(h)	Is often easily distracted by extraneous stimuli	Is not distracted by extraneous stimuli (maintains focus on an activity not of their own choosing regardless of extraneous stimuli unless directed to change focus by someone in a position of authority)
(i)	Is often forgetful in daily activities	Is not forgetful

HYPERACTIVITY

	Symptom	Normal
(a)	Often fidgets with hands or feet or squirms in seat	Sits still for extended time
(b)	Often leaves seat in classroom or in other situations in which remaining seated is expected	Remains seated in classroom as expected

(continues)

(continued)

Symptom	Normal
(c) Often runs about or climbs excessively in situations in which it is inappropriate (in adolescents or adults, may be limited to subjective feelings of restlessness)	Sits still
(d) Often has difficulty playing or engaging in leisure activities quietly	Engages in leisure activities quietly
(e) Is often "on the go" or often acts as if "driven by a motor"	Normal activity level is low to medium
(f) Often talks excessively	Talks when appropriate

IMPULSIVITY

Symptom	Normal
(g) Often blurts out answers before questions have been completed	Waits for questions to be completed before answering
(h) Often has difficulty awaiting turn	Waits his or her turn
(i) Often interrupts or intrudes on others (e.g., butts into conversations or games)	Waits to be invited into conversations and games

Based on the expectations of "normal," what does this sound like to you? It may just be me, but this sounds like a schoolteacher's dream student. This "normal" child sits still for extended periods of time, speaks when spoken to, is patient, and doesn't lose or forget things. The "normal" child is even quiet when engaging in leisure activities. The best part of this for the teacher is that this "normal" child maintains focus on anything they are directed to do until they are directed to do something else.

It's no wonder that ADHD is usually diagnosed at age seven and a half. By this time the child has entered second grade, and the expectations are set. Teachers typically have thirty or more students in a classroom and a lot of material to cover. That would be possible if every student fit the description above of "normal." So the kids that are the furthest from this idealized description of the perfect student are singled out as being the problem. It seems that there is no attempt to question the system that expects young children to sit still and study attentively all day, every day.

The teacher, wanting to help the child who is not in step with the good students in the class, indicates to an administrator or a parent that this child may have a disorder. This is usually done in a formalized meeting around a table full of teachers, school counselors, and administrators. It can be pretty intimidating. The parent or parents are bombarded with tales of the child's problem behaviors, missing assignments, and other proof that there is indeed a problem. A suggestion is made that perhaps it isn't bad parenting. Perhaps there is a medical explanation. The parents usually agree that the child should see a doctor as soon as possible. They are then assured that once the child has a diagnosis, the school will be much more able to help the child.

Many of us can see something of ourselves in the list of symptoms used to diagnose ADHD. However, the criteria are more stringent than that. A diagnosis of ADHD must be based on more than just a list of behaviors. The condition must also cause impairment in two or more settings such as home and school. Since the DSM doesn't offer a definition of "impairment," we'll fall back on this definition found online at *www.thefreedictionary.com* as a point of reference:

> Impairment: The condition of being unable to perform as a consequence of physical or mental unfitness; "reading disability"; "hearing impairment"

Based on the requirement of impairment in two or more settings, it's easy to see why ADHD has traditionally been considered a childhood disorder. The impairments are usually related to expectations of behavior and performance in school. Since schools are dealing with so many children in a single classroom, they simply work better when all the children are on the same program and no one child requires greater-than-average attention. When school activities come home in the form of homework, the impairment comes home, too. Once we're no longer students, the "disorder" seems to go away. But did the underlying condition really go away? Was a side benefit of graduation a cure from ADHD?

Let's say, for example, that a man with ADHD is impaired at home and at work. At home the impairment is related to paying bills on time. The task is boring and so he puts it off and the bills stack up. Then one day he discovers online bill pay. Since he enjoys his computer, the task is quick and easy, and he now pays his bills on time. Since the impairment no longer exists at home, is he cured?

Another criterion required for a diagnosis is "clinically significant impairment" in social, academic, or occupational functioning. The DSM doesn't provide a definition of clinically significant impairment, but it is safe to assume that "clinically significant" is being used in comparison to "statistically significant." For example, a 5-point difference in IQ may be statistically significant in a study, but it wouldn't be considered clinically significant since we wouldn't expect a 5-point difference in IQ to have a profound effect on functioning. Clinical significance requires subjective judgment on which "impairments" are important and which are not. While one person may consider an impairment clinically significant, another with the same level of functioning may disagree on the level of impairment.

It seems unlikely that a true disorder would be cured or eliminated by online bill pay or graduation from school. It is also troublesome to have a disorder defined by a subjective measure of impairment, particularly if the impairment is related to a situation that is temporary. I propose that the underlying condition is still there, but the negative aspects of some of the traits only surface under certain conditions.

NOT ALL DISTRESS OR DIFFERENCE IS MENTAL DISORDER

These people, my people, are different. They do experience some distress and they are impaired in some situations. That does not equal mental disorder. Stephanie Tolan has a beautiful story called "Is It a Cheetah?" which can be found on her website *www.stephanietolan. com*. In the story she uses the cheetah as a metaphor for children with different abilities. She explains acts of lashing out or empty-eyed staring as expressions of frustration, comparing them to a cheetah in captivity throwing itself at the bars of its cage or giving up. She compares the cheetah cage at a zoo to the classroom. This environment doesn't give them the opportunity to show what they are really capable of, so they are not recognized as special, gifted students, and they may be misunderstood as not really trying or even disabled. If this sounds a lot like ADHD, you are beginning to see the light.

There are statistically significant differences that aren't considered disorders such as giftedness. On the scale of intelligence, the bottom 2 percent are considered mentally retarded and therefore subject to a diagnosis of mental disorder. However, the top 2 percent are considered mentally gifted and not subject to a diagnosis of mental disorder. The difference between the two is the expected outcome. Mental retardation is expected to produce less-than-desirable outcomes while giftedness is expected to produce better-than-average outcomes.

It's understandable that intense people would be under consideration as disordered when viewed by people looking for mental disorder. They are different. But, as we see in the example of mentally gifted persons, different doesn't necessarily mean disordered.

Neurodiversity

A new concept of neurodiversity proposes that differences in neurological development in humans is just as important to the health of the human race as biodiversity is to the health of an ecosystem. Neurodiversity takes into account differences in the way different people process information including sound, textures, light, images, and even movement. Although the concept of neurodiversity is associated with a particular view of autism, it applies as well to intensity.

Differences in the way the senses take in information and the way that information is processed in the brain and nervous system make certain types of people better able to adapt to certain environments. The typical school environment is well suited for nonintense people. A preference for convergent or linear thinking (thinking in a straight line with only one possible right answer) makes schools an uncomfortable place for the divergent or nonlinear-thinking brain (spontaneous, free-flowing, and capable of holding many possible solutions) so common in intense people. In this way the values of the society, which control the values in the environment, end up being the determining factor in whether an intense type of neurology is considered a disorder or a gift. Most of our society is congruent with the value system found in the schools; however, there are some pretty important areas where a more intense neurology is a huge advantage. Those who are successful in those areas, such as entrepreneurs, CEOs, inventors, and artists, are likely to be intense.

Asynchronous Development

Hidden behind the concept of impairment is a concept of normal development. Someone who doesn't display the same level of development as their peers in a particular area may be considered impaired, but this view doesn't take asynchronous development into consideration. Asynchronous development is uneven development of intellectual, physical, and/or emotional abilities. The measure of normal development is based on what the average child is capable of at a certain age. A normal five-year-old has a certain range of intellectual, emotional, and physical abilities. An intellectually gifted five-year-old is more likely to perform above grade level intellectually. Gifted children are also more likely to be out of sync in emotional and physical development. A gifted five-year-old may be performing at the intellectual level of a seven-year-old, the physical level of a five-year-old, and the emotional level of a three-year-old. The traditional definition of "gifted" focuses on intelligence and measures of IQ. While the traditional definition of gifted doesn't cover all types of giftedness we now recognize, such as creative genius, the characteristic of asynchronous development still seems to apply.

I look at it like the developmental timelines I see in different species. A puppy takes a week or two to begin walking and can be weaned onto solid food at six to eight weeks. A human takes about a year to begin walking and starts solid food within a few months. That's a drastic difference and perhaps not the best example, but I think you get the idea. A human, who is more complex than a puppy, takes longer to develop. The same seems to be true of humans of different complexities. A less complex person may develop fully by age fifteen. A more complex person may continue to develop for an additional fifteen or thirty years, or perhaps they may never stop developing. So while the intellect is developing, the emotional and physical development may lag behind. In another person the emotional development may be first while the intellectual and physical development catches up later.

The concepts of asynchronous development and neurodiversity caution us to be careful not to label normal human differences as disorders or impairments.

THE DSM IS FALLIBLE

We can see that the DSM changes over time but few people are aware of the extent to which it changes. It is created and maintained by committee and is influenced by changing societal norms, which seems like the best way to keep the manual current. However, a look back at previous diagnosable disorders may provide a more accurate look at the dangers of this type of system to identify disorders.

Runaway Reaction of Childhood

In 1968 the DSM-II identified an interesting disorder called the "runaway reaction of childhood." Individuals with this disorder "characteristically escape from threatening situations by running away from home for a day or more without permission. Typically they are immature and timid, and feel rejected at home, inadequate, and friendless. They often steal furtively."

Marital Maladjustment

Here's a really good one. According to current marital statistics, 50 percent of all couples would eventually fall into this disorder: marital maladjustment. The DSM-II describes those with marital maladjustment disorder as "individuals who are psychiatrically normal but who have significant conflicts or maladjustments in marriage."

Homosexuality

Homosexuality was considered a mental disorder in the DSM until the sixth printing of the DSM-II in 1973. After the gay rights movement began, there were organized protests at APA conferences, which eventually forced the APA to reconsider homosexuality as a psychiatric disorder. This excerpt from the APA's position statement for the proposed removal of homosexuality clarifies the basis for the argument:

> For a mental or psychiatric condition to be considered a psychiatric disorder, it must either regularly cause subjective distress, or regularly be associated with some generalized impairment in social effectiveness or functioning. With the exception of homosexuality (and perhaps some of the other sexual deviations when in mild form, such as voyeurism), all of the other mental disorders in DSM-II fulfill either of these two criteria. While one may argue that the personality disorders are an exception, on reflection it is clear that it is inappropriate to make a diagnosis of a personality disorder merely because of the presence of certain typical personality traits which cause no subjective distress or impairment in social functioning. Clearly homosexuality, per se, does not meet the requirements for a psychiatric disorder since, as noted above, many homosexuals are quite sat-

isfied with their sexual orientation and demonstrate no generalized impairment in social effectiveness or functioning.

The only way that homosexuality could therefore be considered a psychiatric disorder would be the criteria of failure to function heterosexually, which is considered optimal in our society and by many members of our profession. However, if failure to function optimally in some important area of life as judged by either society or the profession is sufficient to indicate the presence of a psychiatric disorder, then we will have to add to our nomenclature the following conditions: celibacy (failure to function optimally sexually), revolutionary behavior (irrational defiance of social norms), religious fanaticism (dogmatic and rigid adherence to religious doctrine), racism (irrational hatred of certain groups), vegetarianism (unnatural avoidance of carnivorous behavior), and male chauvinism (irrational belief in the inferiority of women).

■ ■ ■

As these examples demonstrate, the DSM has flaws. For the ADHD diagnosis, the criteria rely entirely on observable symptoms and subjective interpretations of the distress caused by them. We could use a similar argument to the one made for removing the homosexuality diagnosis to consider the removal of ADHD as a disorder. Many intense people are quite satisfied with their lives, including the differences in the way their brains work. The majority of the "distress" reported in children with an ADHD diagnosis is the distress of the teacher. That just doesn't count. However, I recognize that humans experience distress sometimes. I will argue that distress is a perfectly normal human condition that intense people feel more commonly. While consulting a mental health professional can help reduce distress, the presence of distress by itself doesn't constitute a mental disorder. Even the argument to remove homosexuality from the DSM as a disorder allowed that some people who consider themselves homosexual may experience distress. If that distress is severe, they can and should seek treatment, but the problem is the distress, not necessarily the homosexuality.

If we discard the condition of distress, we are left with the condition of impairment. In this case, as in the case with homosexuality, the impairment is based on a societal norm that is more a matter of personality and environment than it is a matter of disorder. While some environments such as school make it seem as though intense people are impaired, other environments make it seem as though they are uniquely gifted. If there isn't impairment and there isn't distress, there isn't disorder.

In the DSM-5 there are changes to both the symptoms and the age of onset of ADHD. Symptoms must only have been present before age twelve. In prior versions it was age seven. Also the list of symptoms was modified to include an adult version of each so that it will be easier to diagnose adults.

The changes planned by the APA in the DSM-5 that make it easier to diagnose ADHD are suspect to say the least. These changes are taking place in spite of a plea from a previous chairman of the taskforce that created the DSM-IV. Dr. Allen Frances pleads for an end to this practice in an article titled "It's Not Too Late to Save 'Normal.'" He identifies ADHD as one of the areas where the taskforce made the biggest errors:

> Our panel tried hard to be conservative and careful but inadvertently contributed to three false "epidemics"—attention deficit disorder, autism and childhood bipolar disorder. Clearly, our net was cast too wide and captured many "patients" who might have been far better off never entering the mental health system.

Frances continues with a concern that the proposed DSM-5 "is filled with suggestions that would multiply our mistakes and extend the reach of psychiatry dramatically deeper into the ever-shrinking domain of the normal."

Dr. Frances attributes the move toward an increase in diagnosing normal people as disordered to inadvertent mistakes made by the panel trying hard to be "conservative and careful." But we have to wonder what kind of influence the pharmaceutical companies continue to have over the decision-making process, particularly when we see the proposed changes in the DSM-5.

TOO COMMON TO BE A DISORDER

The DSM-IV states the prevalence of ADHD as 3 to 5 percent. Based on more recent studies, this prevalence rate is not accurate today. According to the CDC (Centers for Disease Control and Prevention), the prevalence of parent-reported ADHD averaged 9.5 percent in 2007. In a 2007 study of the prevalence of ADHD in children age four to seventeen by state, the results varied from a low of 5.6 percent in Nevada to a high of 15.6 percent in North Carolina. These results were compared with a study completed in 2003. The prevalence has grown by 22 percent in four years.

The National Institute of Mental Health (NIMH) lists the prevalence rate of other disorders at a lower rate. Schizophrenia and autism spectrum disorder are each found in less than 1 percent of the population. Obsessive-compulsive disorder is also in the 1 percent range. This is compared to a reported prevalence of ADHD in 9 percent of children and 4.1 percent of adults.

Going back to the DSM-III, ADHD is described as a common childhood disorder with a nearly 3 percent prevalence rate. If 3 percent is common, what is 9 percent? With the changes in the DSM-5, the prevalence is expected to increase. At what point do we look at a pattern of behaviors as within the normal range? If it isn't 9 percent, is it 15 percent, or perhaps 30 percent?

There is no need to explain or label behavior that is within the norm, only that which lies outside the norm. And it should be pretty far outside the norm to qualify as a mental disorder. Statistically speaking, it should be at least two standard deviations from the norm. In English, that means that it should be either in the bottom 2 to 2.5 percent or in the top 2 to 2.5 percent, leaving about 95 to 96 percent of the population to fall within statistic normality.

A report published in 2003 on the concerns of overdiagnosis of ADHD in school-age children indicates that statistical rarity is the only method by which to measure developmental deviance:

> In fact, definitions of some disorders—including ADHD—are reliant on the concept of *statistical rarity*, or what is sometimes referred to as *developmental deviance*. Consider the case of mental retardation vis-à-vis intelligence. Mental retardation (the condition) is defined by intelligence (the construct) that is measured to be at least two standard deviations below the population mean. While some individuals may have low intelligence, only those whose intelligence is significantly developmentally deviant (i.e., statistically rare) are considered disordered. The diagnosis of ADHD is conceptually akin to that of mental retardation in that the definition of both disorders relies on the concept of developmental deviance. As with intelligence, the hallmark symptoms of ADHD (impulsivity, hyperactivity, and inattention) exist in all children to some degree, but ADHD is said to exist only when the behaviors are expressed to an extreme or statistically rare degree.

> Given that the definition of ADHD is based on statistical rarity, only a limited number of children can qualify as having the disorder. As in the case of mental retardation, the ADHD

prevalence estimate was set at 3 percent to 5 percent, which restricts the disorder to those children whose ADHD-related behavioral characteristics are approximately two standard deviations away from the mean. The 3 percent to 5 percent estimate may constitute a liberal estimate because, as with mental retardation, statistical rarity is only one of several criteria for the diagnosis.

If the statistical rarity criterion holds, prevalence rates of greater than 3 to 5 percent cannot occur. Actually a statistical rarity would have to be two standard deviations from the mean. Using this kind of measure, roughly 95 percent of people should fall within the two standard deviations. The remaining 5 percent would fall equally to either side. So if we are trying to determine what an abnormal level of attention is according to this measure, about 2.5 percent would fall in the lowest end of the spectrum, which may be considered developmentally deviant.

If our current rates of diagnosis are four times the highest rate that could be possible given the criteria, what is causing the epidemic? If there is no epidemic, it must be something else.

THERE IS *NO* PROOF OF DISORDER

Even though we have ample proof that ADHD is at least overdiagnosed, we still haven't proven that it doesn't exist. On the other hand, I question if anyone can prove that it does exist. There are no objective tests that prove the existence of ADHD or any other psychiatric disorder. The diagnoses are all based on subjective measures. That fact alone doesn't prove that they don't exist, but it should be cause to use greater scrutiny.

Dr. Sami Timimi, who has authored several books on child psychiatry, contends that there is no proof of ADHD. While there have been attempts to identify objective tests and measures of ADHD as a disorder, none exist to date. Even in seemingly objective neuroimaging studies, he warns that

> researchers have yet to compare un-medicated children diagnosed with ADHD with an age-matched control group. Sample sizes in these studies have been small and have produced a variety of inconsistent results. In no study were the brains considered clinically abnormal, nor is it possible to work out whether any differences seen are caused by (rather than being the causes of) different styles of thinking, or are the result of the medication the children had taken.

He also identifies an interesting fact: that prevalence rates of ADHD vary considerably, from less than half of a percent to 26 percent in studies because of the uncertainty of description.

I'll be the first to agree that there is something different about the people typically diagnosed with ADHD. However, if the symptoms can be better explained by something else, and if that different explanation makes better outcomes possible, we should be certain to explore that as a possibility. Doctors, by virtue of the Hippocratic oath, should be bound to consider an alternate explanation.

IF NOT DISORDER, THEN WHAT?

There were once six blind men who were asked to describe an elephant. The one who touched the ear said it was like a fan. The one who touched the trunk said it was like a large pipe. The others who felt only the belly or the tail or the leg or the tusk had different explanations. When they were told that they were each right and that they had each described a portion of the elephant, they still couldn't fathom the entire beast.

Like the story of the blind men and the elephant, the descriptions of the underlying condition responsible for ADHD fall short when offered from a limited view. The underlying condition is one of intensity. The description in the DSM of ADHD is limited by its purpose of identifying the disorder by the negative aspects of intensity. This lack of understanding of the underlying condition of intensity contributes to both misdiagnosis and a lack of education about and healthy development of intensity.

Every natural human trait can be viewed by either its negative or positive side. In truth a trait is the combination of all its aspects, negative and positive. If you can think of a trait that seems to belong to only one side, you're not thinking of a trait but of an aspect of a larger thing. For example, inattention is not a trait, but an aspect of the larger category of attention. On the one end of the spectrum of attention is inattention, and on the other is hyperfocus.

Instead of experiencing just the middle range of these traits, people who are often diagnosed with ADHD experience more of the range. They go from inattention to those things that are not interesting to hyperfocus on those things that are interesting to them. It's natural for any human to pay closer attention to something that's interesting and less attention to something that is not as interesting. However, when a subgroup of people have a greater range, we then make the low end of the range and the high end of the range symptoms of a disorder. If we consider the trait of activity, on one end we have lethargy and on the other we have both impulsivity and hyperactivity. It's interesting to me that we accept lethargy as within the range of normal, while the other end of the spectrum is considered abnormal.

If we concentrate only on the perceived negatives of having a greater range, we're missing half the picture. With a greater range of attention, we are never inattentive; we are always taking in more than others. We have the ability to take in information that is going on around us that others screen out. This has been described as missing the "space bubble" that others use to screen out unimportant stimuli. But when the thing we are attending to is of great importance to us, we have a super space bubble. Nothing else matters. We can stay on a single subject or activity for a very long time without noticing anything else going on around us. This is then called hyperfocus and considered a symptom. Instead of looking at the positive side of this greater-than-average ability to attend to a single thing, we say that this is evidence of being "stuck."

By concentrating on the negative interpretation of each of the traits, we are ultimately convinced that we have a problem. The worst part of this is that we are never encouraged to develop the positive side. It becomes a self-fulfilling prophecy. We see only the negative, we concentrate on the negative, we have it pointed out to us on a regular basis, and we become only the negative.

If the description of intensity on the following pages better fits your experience of the world, and if it helps you to understand yourself and your potential better, then use that description in place of "ADHD."

For ADHD professionals, know that intense people are becoming self-aware. A psychiatrist, psychologist, school counselor, coach, or pediatrician who has a solid understanding of intensity will always be valued. This doesn't mean the end of your involvement with these people. It's only the beginning of what should be a much more satisfying journey together, one where you can actually offer some help in development of their inherent gifts and a better understanding of their distress.

Important Points for the Impatient

- There is no proof of ADHD as a disorder. There exists no objective method of diagnosis for ADHD. Even the neuroimaging studies have failed to produce adequate tests with comparisons to "normal" brains in subjects of the same age.

- If there is no proof of disorder, there is no cure offered, and the treatment used to manage the condition can be deadly, we have to look for another explanation. If there is an alternate explanation that offers a better outcome, in good conscience doctors should be required to consider it. Adherence to the Hippocratic oath should require them to consider it. We should consider it for ourselves.

2

What Is Intensity?

"Ode to Intensity"
For lighting the stars in the autumn night sky
For softening the green grass on which I lie
For painting the sunset with colors of heart
As the light of the sun and the sky tear apart

For filling the music with brilliance uplifting
And smiles regardless of sands of time sifting
For showing me wingless and grounded to fly
And for lighting the stars in the autumn night sky
                                    —STEPHAN PATTERSON

There are many ways to look at intensity. Many doctors present the unique combinations of traits as a form of mental or physical disability. They speak fluently in brain scans and pharmaceuticals. They enjoy identifying aspects of the brain, the body, or socialization that indicate a departure from "normal" in very intense people. This is, of course, one way of looking at it. The problem with this view is that it defines a person as sick and seeks to find cures. One could then be convinced to try different medications, counseling, labels, etc. The bottom line is that this approach requires one to believe that she is deficient as a human being.

What if that perception is entirely wrong? What if you are a completely normal human being? Differences don't necessarily mean illness.

Have you heard the story of the ugly duckling? The poor little fellow was hatched with a group of lovely and proper ducklings. By comparison he was a terrible disappointment. He had grey feathers instead of yellow, his quack was more like a honk, and his only redeeming quality was that he could swim. It turns out that the duckling wasn't ugly, or awkward, or unable to quack. He was a swan. Had that swan remained with the ducks and never met another swan, he may have lived out his life believing himself to be a poor excuse for a duck, being ashamed of his long neck and enormous stature. Instead he found his own kind. In the Hans Christian Andersen version, the ugly duckling flies to the swans thinking they will kill him for his ugliness, his "swan song" of sorts. It's not until he bends his head down, waiting for the first blow, that he sees his reflection in the water and understands that he is one of the swans. The swans greet him warmly, and even the children who had taunted and teased him as an ugly duckling are in awe of his beauty.

Intense people are like the swan. If we don't find our own identity, we are destined to wander the world of ducks thinking of ourselves as disordered. Who are the swans you know? Are they the entrepreneurs, social reform leaders, actors, poets, and artists? Are they scientists and CEOs and authors? Can you see your reflection in them?

KAZIMIERZ DABROWSKI IDENTIFIES "SUPER-STIMULATABILITY"

Many years ago there was a doctor in Poland who specialized in swans like us. Kazimierz Dabrowski not only lived through World War I as a young person, but also survived World War II as the Polish culture was condemned by the Nazis. Education and the arts went underground as Germany attempted to destroy the Polish culture. Dr. Dabrowski sheltered Jews and was imprisoned by the Nazis. Even after the war he was imprisoned by the communists because of his strong stance for individual self-determination. His focus of study was gifted and creative people.

Given the social circumstances at the time and the sentiments of Nazi Germany toward the arts and intellectual pursuits, his interest in gifted and creative people makes a lot of sense. Dabrowski found that gifted and creative people share a profound difference from others in that they have a more intense experience of life. The word he used to name the intensities translates most closely to "super-stimulatability." Most English translations use the term "overexcitability." There are those that object to the term because as soon as you say over, you imply that it's too much. Super has a better connotation. To avoid the whole thing, I use the term "intensity." What it means is that given the same amount of stimulus, these people react more than others. If the stimulus is physical, such as a pin prick, the normal person may flinch while the intense person may flinch a bit more. The stimulus causes a greater reaction in the intense person because the stimulus is intensified for them. It is not a case of overreaction; it has to do with amplification of the stimulus. This is an important distinction—really important. It is perhaps the most misunderstood thing about intense people. Again, intense people are not overreacting. They are reacting appropriately for the amount of stimulus they receive. Their receptors seem to be more sensitive because their nervous system amplifies the input.

Dabrowski believed that these intense gifted and creative people were capable of advanced development, not in spite of the intensities, but because of them. The heightened experiences including pain, stress, and discomfort cause these people to have greater opportunities for what he called positive disintegration, or the falling apart of a person's view of reality. He understood that a positive side to disintegration exists in the building of a new view of reality at a higher level. This is a natural growth process. If you think about the person you were in your twenties or earlier, and then think about the person you are now, you'll see a difference. Your attitudes, beliefs, and view of the world have changed. These changes happened when your view of the world no longer worked. You had no choice but to let it fall apart and rebuild it so that you could handle the situation that was intolerable in your old view of the world.

Dabrowski recognized that super-stimulatability produces more intense moments, which create more opportunities to go through a similar growth process where the worldview seems to fall apart and then reorganize itself at a higher level of understanding about reality. I agree that an intense nature provides the possibility of advanced development, but that's just the beginning. When intensities are recognized, developed, and employed in the right way, they provide an almost unfair advantage in creating and reaching the most grandiose goals in life.

Identifying intensity in yourself is difficult. If I've always lived in my own skin, how would I know what it feels like to be inside someone else's skin? How would I know if my perception of a stimulus is stronger than someone else's? I don't! That's a part of the problem. In fact the most common reaction is to assume that other people feel and sense things exactly as I do. I then imagine that they have better control over the expression of the reaction. This is not only common but also a big reason that intense people assume themselves to be disordered. Instead of the intense person having a deficit in the ability to control their reactions, they have a nervous system that intensifies the stimuli.

THE FIVE INTENSITIES

There are five areas where intensity shows up. Dabrowski calls the five intensities sensual, imaginational, psychomotor, intellectual, and emotional. My list of intensities varies only in that I use the term "creative intensity" rather than "imaginational." This not only better describes the intensity, but also enables a nifty little acronym for the intensities, SPICE, since the intensities are the spice of life:

S   sensual

P   psychomotor

I   intellectual

C   creative

E   emotional

The list of traits of each intensity is not complete, nor can it be, because intensities are endlessly complex. Also a person with an intensity may not have all the symptoms on the list. This is not a diagnostic tool. It's intended to give you a flavor of the intensity. If a few of the items on a list sound familiar to you, you may have that intensity to some degree.

Sensual Intensity

The five senses are really perceived through the nervous system. Although the eyes, ears, nose, tongue, and skin seem to be the source of the sensations, the input from each of them has to pass through a network of communication channels and on to the brain before the sensation registers. The differences in sensual intensity are differences of degree. Everyone has senses, but those with sensual intensity have those senses amplified.

A person with sensual intensity traits

(a) finds loud places or bright lights uncomfortable.

(b) is often bothered by tight clothing, tags that rub against the skin, or seams in socks; shops by feel for clothing, bedding, or anything that touches the skin; is drawn to softness.

(c) complains of pain in situations that others find tolerable (e.g., dental exams, heat or cold, or muscle tension); regularly takes pain relievers.

(d) may recoil when touched if the touch is not gentle or if light enough to tickle. (Children may brace themselves when adults hug them.)

(e) notices and appreciates beauty in places where others may miss it. (He may be captivated by a beautiful scene in nature or the glistening and swirling of a drop of oil in a rain-soaked street.)

(f) is often visibly affected by a piece of music. (Children may express early preferences for certain types of music or favorite songs.)

(g) may have strong emotional or physical reactions to smells. (While one smell may trigger an immediate nostalgic return to another time and place, another may trigger nausea.)

(h) may be a picky eater with sensitivity to the textures in food. (An adult may have a sensitive palate and appreciate fine foods.)

(i) has a tendency to use alcohol, drugs, or food to soothe the physical discomfort of living.

Psychomotor Intensity

The ADHD version of this is called hyperactivity. This sometimes shows up as a person moving about too much as described in the ADHD list of symptoms. More often in adults, this psychomotor intensity is internalized. It can be a feeling of restlessness that leaks out in a need to keep some part of the body moving. Sometimes if the body can't keep the pace, the mind will start moving really fast. Psychomotor intensity is a predisposition toward or a preference for action.

A person with psychomotor intensity traits

(a) often fidgets, taps hands or feet, or squirms in seat (e.g., Jimmy legs, hand wringing, pencil tapping).

(b) is often restless in situations that require remaining seated for long periods of time such as air travel or long meetings. She may pace when on the telephone. (Children may have trouble staying seated in a classroom.)

(c) often talks excessively and blurts or interrupts others. (She may answer a question before it has been completed, complete other people's sentences, or not yield the floor when a point has already been made.)

(d) is often impatient, as shown by feeling restless when waiting for others and wanting to move faster than others, wanting people to get to the point, speeding while driving, and cutting into traffic to go faster than others.

(e) is uncomfortable doing things slowly and systematically and often rushes through activities or tasks.

(f) tends to act without pausing long enough to think it through (e.g., makes impulse purchases, walks off a job, commits to a relationship after a brief time).

(g) has multiple projects going at the same time and has enough energy for all of them.

(h) takes on tasks and projects that might intimidate others. She may attempt things that are usually left to professionals such as a remodeling project or rebuilding an engine.

(i) may use caffeine or nicotine to modulate energy.

Intellectual Intensity

Intellectual intensity reveals the ability to extend both sides of the attentional spectrum. When interested in something, an intense person can focus on it for an extended amount of time and not notice other things going on in the environment. This fascination with a subject can last for hours or days or years. Intellectually intense people crave intellectual stimulation. They devour books and newspapers. They can spend hours researching on the Internet. Time seems to stand still until they realize that they've been reading for hours. This fascination with learning and collecting information is usually in a few select subjects, although I've known some who seem to follow so many subjects it seems as though they are intensely interested in everything. The flip side of this intense intellectual pursuit is that there is no tolerance for subjects that are not interesting. This extends into performing tasks that aren't interesting, which provides fodder for psychologists and psychiatrists to label a person as having a deficit of attention.

A person with intellectual intensity traits

(a) often fails to give close attention to details, makes careless mistakes, and has difficulty sustaining attention in tasks that are deemed uninteresting or unimportant.

(b) misplaces objects necessary for tasks or activities (e.g., school assignments, pencils, books, tools, wallets, keys, paperwork, eyeglasses, cell phones, or the remote).

 (c) often has difficulty organizing tasks and activities and/or has spurts of intense organization.

(d) notices everything or focuses exclusively on only one thing (e.g., notices children playing in peripheral vision while driving, fails to notice a person talking to them while concentrating on something).

(e) has a constant need for information (e.g., newspapers, piles of books everywhere, hours on the Internet).

(f) is capable of extended periods of focus on a subject or project to the exclusion of all else.

(g) displays natural curiosity and a love of learning that doesn't stop with formal education.

(h) is adept with abstract reasoning and divergent thinking.

 (i) may possess a sense of perfectionism that may create frustration and in some cases fear of failure.

Creative Intensity

One of the clues to recognizing creative intensity is a tendency to daydream. This intensity is sometimes called imaginational intensity because the strongest characteristic is a healthy imagination. These people have not only a great imagination, but also a need to create. Creativity is like a therapy for them, soothing and healing effortlessly. Whether they are creating works of art, works of industry, or crafts, the amount of time spent in creative endeavors is directly proportional to their health and well-being.

A person with creative intensity traits

(a) often does not seem to listen when spoken to directly (her mind seems elsewhere; she seems spacey).

(b) is often easily distracted by extraneous stimuli (stimuli can trigger an imaginational journey).

(c) demonstrates a preference for starting projects with less energy at the finish. Unfinished projects can be found in closets, garages, and sometimes taking over whole rooms.

(d) has a vivid imagination and love of fantasy. In children there may be imaginary friends. In adults there may be a love of novels or fantasy games.

(e) has a tendency to give inanimate objects human traits (e.g., giving a car a name and an imagined personality).

(f) has a need to create in order to achieve a sense of inner peace. (Any type of creative endeavor from macramé to oil painting provides a sense of physical and emotional relief.)

(g) prefers the unusual and unique and tends to relate events in a "most interesting first" order instead of sequential order.

(h) has a healthy grandiosity. Ideas and planned endeavors are not limited by what others believe is reasonable or realistic. She is happy to dream up and take on larger-than-life projects.

(i) has a low tolerance for boredom and will fill boring time with imagination.

(j) may experience nightmares, worry, and anxiety over imagined threats and problems.

Emotional Intensity

Emotional intensity is easily recognized both in someone else and in yourself. If people often tell you to calm down or lighten up, or if you have been dubbed a drama queen, a hothead, or too sensitive, you may be emotionally intense. Emotional intensity is the one intensity that brings more people to therapy or coaching than anything else. This intensity has the biggest impact on your experience of life.

A person with emotional intensity traits

(a) is often driven by fluctuating moods with rapid changes. (This is different from bipolar disorder in that the mood changes are more frequent and not as long lasting.)

(b) experiences intense and seemingly unpredictable emotions, causing some difficulty in social interactions. The complexity of this intensity is not well understood by others, creating a sense of uncertainty for others and a sense of separation for the emotionally intense person.

(c) may feel anxiety due to sensitivity and increased perceptivity. An awareness of the extent of the differences between one's self and the majority of society creates the feeling of not quite fitting in.

(d) may have anger-management issues. These are misunderstood and don't respond well to typical anger-management interventions.

(e) may suffer extreme and debilitating depression.

(f) expresses enthusiasm that gets noticed. Gestures and facial expressions are bigger than normal, seem too enthusiastic, and sometimes draw ridicule.

(g) is sensitive to animals and anyone or anything seen as help-less. He is likely to take in stray animals or go above and beyond to help others.

(h) senses the emotions of others. He detects nuances of body language and reads the emotional field of others. Incongru-ence sensed in others can cause distress. He is susceptible to taking on the emotional field of others in his immediate physical surroundings.

(i) has a special need for safety and comfort. A tendency to need safety and comfort is counteracted by a tendency to need stimulation and excitement. (Safety is a requirement for future emotional development.)

■ ■ ■

Do you see yourself in the reflection? In the last chapter I challenged you to hold off on deciding if there is such a thing as ADHD until you heard an alternate explanation of the underlying condition. Do the intensities sound familiar to you? If so, I invite you to consider intensity as a better, more complete explanation of the way you are. It's an opportunity to leave disorder behind by understanding your true nature and developing your intensities instead of trying to deny or suppress them.

Most intense people were never taught how to handle their in-tensity. There was usually at least one intense parent, but that parent was most likely focused on helping the child fit in. Having a good understanding of intensity, the unique way it manifests in your life, and how to manage it are subjects normally left untouched. But hav-ing that information can have a profound positive effect on your experience of life. That's the purpose of this book.

INTENSITY: GIFT OR DISORDER?

In a manner of speaking, you were told about your intensities if and when you were diagnosed with ADHD. And with that focus, the immediate reaction was to try to remedy your weaknesses. You may have finally understood why you have always had trouble keeping things organized or getting the bills paid on time. What's more, you had an explanation that meant that you weren't at fault. It may have come as a relief. The options available to you with this view of yourself are focused on limiting the damage of your weaknesses. You may learn coping mechanisms, begin taking medications, develop some new skills, or find organizational or time-management aids. You may have therapy or coaching to help you recognize your weaknesses and deal with the emotional blow of finding out that you have a disorder. What all these actions have in common is that they are based on weaknesses.

We now know that it's pretty much a waste of time to try to fix weaknesses. Sure, you can make some progress, with a lot of effort. But one thing is sure: You'll never be great at something that is a natural weakness no matter how much time and energy you spend trying to fix it. I want to clarify two things here. First, a weakness in an area of knowledge is definitely worth addressing. Things that can be learned are not in the same category as natural strengths and weaknesses. Second, some of the areas you may have considered weaknesses may turn out to be strengths when you better understand your intensity. There are several books worth a read if you're interested in this. Research done at the Gallup Organization on the differences between average and successful businesses and managers turned up some surprising results, which led to the book *First, Break All the Rules* by Marcus Buckingham and Curt Coffman. One of the most interesting things Buckingham and Coffman found about the more successful businesses and managers is that they spent more time and energy developing their strongest people than their weakest. What's more, they didn't spend much time working on weaknesses of even the strongest team members. They concentrated on developing the strengths.

After years of conventional wisdom saying that you have to help your people develop where they are weakest, this came as a surprise. It turns out that time spent developing natural talents into strengths pays off much more than time spent overcoming weaknesses. This book was followed by *Now, Discover Your Strengths* and finally *Go Put Your Strengths to Work*. These are worth reading, particularly in terms of how to use your specific strengths in any job you currently have. It turns out that you don't necessarily have to start all over again with a new career path. For our purposes the research provides a refreshing view of the strengths and weaknesses of intense people and leads to a novel approach.

The common view of ADHD is nothing more than a list of weaknesses. Conventional wisdom makes this list of weaknesses into a disorder, thereby making the people who display these weaknesses patients. It takes the flawed logic that organizations use to concentrate on the weaknesses of employees and ups the ante by making the weaknesses a disorder.

Concentrating on the weaknesses not only doesn't help much, but also actually causes harm. The very fact that a group of people who are uniquely gifted are fooled into spending their time focusing on their weaknesses is no less than criminal. This focus prevents the development of their natural talents. First, drugging ourselves into being "normal" robs us of the gifts that allow us to be spectacular. Second, because the weaknesses are so closely related to the natural talents, we are pushed in the opposite direction. Due to fear and shame of the weakness, we are encouraged to suppress the intensity entirely instead of developing the natural talent inherent in it.

Concentrating instead on developing the intensity, even though it is related to the weakness, produces the best results. Our intensities are our strengths. They are what make us special and different and capable of amazing things. But there's a cost associated with shifting our focus to the strengths. This cannot be done while still holding on to the concept of disorder. That's the price. You can no longer blame your forgetfulness, hyperactivity, impulsiveness, or lack of organization on ADHD. You can't hide behind a disorder. I say this with a full understanding of how difficult that may be. The ADHD label provides support, an easy way for others to understand your challenges, and quite possibly the only explanation so far that left you with your dignity intact. This radical notion that you don't have a disorder threatens that dignity once again. It's as if I'm telling you that you are to blame for all the failures you've experienced. Far from it! There's a big difference between blame and responsibility. This new view of you as intense, and far from disordered, requires a new relationship with and understanding of responsibility. With new information, you have new ways of responding. The ability to *respond* is the essence of *responsibility*. With a thorough understanding of your intensities, there's an opportunity to develop your strengths and minimize your weaknesses, which wasn't available to you before. You have an opportunity to respond to the new information in a way that provides the greatest possibility for your future.

But how am I to get over my weaknesses, you ask? You're probably not going to get over them. Again, this is worth repeating: You're probably not going to get over your weaknesses. That's the reality. There are three methods of dealing with weaknesses. First, you can find a system that helps, such as a time-management system to effectively plan and carry out those plans. Second, find someone else to do those things that you don't do well and you don't need to do personally. And finally accept that there are some things that are just worth doing poorly or not at all.

You can focus the rest of your life on your weakest areas and perhaps make a little improvement. Or you can pretty much ignore them and concentrate on developing your intensities. You'll probably make about the same amount of improvement in your areas of weakness by developing your intensities, and in some situations you'll make much more progress. The difference is that you won't care about the weaknesses so much if you've developed your strengths, and you'll have a much better time. Honestly, having a well-organized desk is just not that important to me. But having the ability to write this book and be able to share all this with you is the most important thing in my life right now. And it is possible because of the methods I share in this book to develop your intensities and use those to achieve any goal you choose.

Keep in mind that everyone has weaknesses. This method of developing strengths instead of spending precious time on weaknesses is not unique to intense people. It just happens to work better and have a bigger impact for us. That's the beauty of intensity. More of everything!

Important Points for the Impatient

- Differences don't necessarily mean disorder. It's a matter of context, like in the story of the ugly duckling. Intense people are like the swan, and finding that out can change everything.

- Dr. Kazimierz Dabrowski identified five intensities in gifted and creative people. They are sensual, psychomotor, intellectual, creative, and emotional. They are the "SPICE" of life.

- These intensities correspond to the symptoms of ADHD perfectly, except that they identify the whole intensity instead of just focusing on the negative aspects.

- It's a waste of time to focus on your areas of weakness. This has been proven and documented in studies by the Gallup Organization. Concentrating on your weaknesses actually causes more damage.

- Instead of subduing or ignoring your intensities, developing them into strengths will produce the best results and even help to mediate your weaknesses.

3

Practice Foundations

In learning, sadness and enthusiasm live in us at the same time: sadness at being aware that we are losing something we have held on to for a long time, and enthusiasm at the possibility of embracing a new way of being.

—JULIO OLALLA

Throughout this book are practices to help develop the intensities. They're based on foundations borrowed from different disciplines including psychology, ontology, and neuroscience. While you may be familiar with psychology and neuroscience, ontology is foreign to most. Ontology is the study of being. Within the context of coaching, it is the practice of helping people through life transitions and growth and, as a result, relieving human suffering by taking the entire being into consideration. Many of the concepts within this book are derived directly from this discipline, including the internal map of reality (known in ontological coaching as the observer), breakdowns, everything being related to everything, and the witness (known as the observer of the observer). These disciplines contribute to practices that are designed to work with the natural methods of bringing about change. As a result there is very little effort and very big results. We take advantage of the mind being a goal-seeking mechanism by directing it to seek the goals of our choosing instead of the default goals that come with the software. This is based on a different understanding of the software of the entire being, how it works, and how you can master it.

THE BODY AS THE SUBCONSCIOUS MIND

The mind is made up of conscious and subconscious components. But where are they exactly? Are they in different parts of the brain? If so, where's the dividing line? This is a question that has vexed neurobiologists and psychologists for decades.

Dr. Candace Pert was working at the National Institutes of Health when she discovered something amazing. She found molecules within the body that were previously only thought to exist in the brain. What's more, these molecules, called neuropeptides, have been associated with the transmission of emotional information. At this point she realized that the emotional brain could no longer be considered to be isolated to the traditional locations within the brain in our heads. Our bodies have an emotional brain as well. As she tried to isolate these molecules within the body, she found that there are areas with high concentrations of neuropeptides. They are correlated with areas where sensory information is processed. She ultimately found that these molecules of emotion have pathways interrupted by areas she referred to as "hot spots" where the signal is interrupted and filtered. Only a portion of the information is allowed to pass through the hot spots. The result is that sensory information comes into the body and is carried by these molecules of emotion, through the hot spots where they are filtered, and some portion of the information makes its way into consciousness. She finally concluded that the body is actually the unconscious mind.

Take a moment with that. It's likely to turn your ideas upside down. Instead of information coming into your consciousness, and some leaking into your subconscious, it's the other way around. All input comes into the subconscious mind, which is housed in the body, and some leaks into consciousness. It makes perfect sense. That's why you find that there is more information in your subconscious about events your conscious mind doesn't even remember until you're under hypnosis. The subconscious takes it all in. Every event of your life, perhaps even every detail of every event, is held in the subconscious.

Memories are, very literally, stored in the body. There is a massage therapy technique called "Rolfing" based on the work of Dr. Ida Rolf, a biochemist. The intent is to realign the muscles and connective tissue to allow the body to return to a more normal posture, promoting health. From personal accounts told to me, I know that this method of massage often reveals memories and emotional pockets within the body. By pressing on a particular place, a memory is revealed and the resultant emotional outpouring is experienced by the patient. Ultimately, I am told, this creates a psychological healing along with the physical benefits of massage. Again, this makes perfect sense once we realize that the body houses the subconscious mind.

THE GATEKEEPER BETWEEN THE SUBCONSCIOUS AND CONSCIOUS MINDS

Think of the reality of the conscious mind being wrapped in a cocoon. The outside world is only perceived by the five senses. Each of these senses is first stopped and interpreted by the subconscious mind in the body at various gates, or what Dr. Pert called hot spots. The subconscious mind acts as a gatekeeper. At each point it stops the incoming traffic, evaluates it, and either opens the gate or refuses to let the input through. This gatekeeper uses three primary criteria to evaluate input:

1. Does it signal a threat of danger? (Imagine hearing your front door closing when no one else is supposed to be home.)

2. Is it important? (Hey, that looks just like my new car!)

3. Has the conscious mind told the gatekeeper to be on the lookout for it? (Such as when you're looking for your other shoe.)

There is a constant stream of input being sent to your conscious mind from the subconscious mind—the words you're reading, the feel of the book in your hands, etc. At the same time, the subconscious mind may choose to ignore the pressure of your clothes against your skin or the sound of people talking in the background. The whole world is experienced directly only by the subconscious mind! The conscious mind is wrapped in a cocoon of the subconscious mind. This protective cocoon decides what gets to make it into consciousness and what doesn't. The subconscious mind is actually determining what we see and what we miss in the world. It becomes very important now to understand how the subconscious mind determines what gets passed through each gate and what stays out.

THE INTERNAL MAP OF REALITY

As the subconscious mind attempts to organize sensory input, it needs some rules to follow. If everything got through to consciousness, you would be overwhelmed with sensory input to the point of being incapable of functioning. The determination of what to filter out and what to leave in has to have some structure, some criteria. It can't be random. Our gatekeeper must use a map of sorts to make the determinations. And this map can't be static. It has to be flexible, allowing it to change as needed, and it must be custom-built for each person. After all, what's important to me may not be important to you. My subconscious mind, or gatekeeper, has to know the difference, as does yours. If all our filters were identical, we would all have the same experience of reality. We would all notice the same things and have the same reactions. But we're all different, and that means that our gatekeepers use at least slightly different filters. So what are they using to decide?

One of the better explanations of the model used by the subconscious mind was provided by Bill Harris (founder of the Holosync system and Centerpointe, discussed in chapter 5). He proposes that the subconscious mind uses a database of sorts to make the filtering decisions. He calls this database an internal map of reality. As he explains it, we form a miniature map of reality in our minds. Since reality is too complex to store, we have a map that serves as a model. It serves the same purpose as a street map of a territory. It is a small model with a lot of generalizations that allows us to understand the territory at a high level. With a street map we understand that we can't really drive on the little lines. They aren't really roads, but they represent roads. We know that the little triangles that represent campgrounds aren't really big enough to pitch a tent. But the map does serve to orient us to our surroundings and identifies points of interest. Just as a map of a city or countryside allows us to get our bearings while traveling, our internal map of reality allows us to make sense of our experience of the world.

Our inner map of reality contains beliefs, opinions, values, attitudes, and many other forms of understanding the meaning of what we encounter in the real reality. Because we have this map, we are freed from having to evaluate everything each time it is encountered. The map contains generalizations of every idea, concept, value, belief, object, person, and situation it may encounter. It uses this map to decide which bits of input make it past the filters and which stay behind. If the input fits within the existing map, it can then be evaluated in terms of the threat it may present and the importance to the conscious mind. If the input doesn't fit the existing map, it will either be altered to fit the map or it will not be passed along to the conscious mind. As the gatekeeper evaluates input, the determination of what is important and what is threatening is determined by comparing the input against the internal map of reality.

We didn't consciously create the map. It was primarily given to us by our family, culture, and early experiences. By the time we reached the age of reason, the map was almost completely formed. The other really startling thing about this map is that we don't even know that it is controlling everything. Because it is a tool used by the subconscious mind, it is, by definition, outside of our awareness. We are never privy to the filters being applied to the sensory input.

So, what a predicament! Our conscious minds are being spoon-fed information from our subconscious minds. We believe the input we are receiving is an accurate representation of reality. We think that we are actually seeing, hearing, and feeling reality. But in fact, we have been filtering all that input based on a map of reality that we didn't even consciously create. For most people, this is where the story ends. This is exactly how they go through their lives, never being aware of the illusion they are living.

The Conscious Mind's Effect on the Map

One of the best things about this situation is that the subconscious mind is very willing to take direction from the conscious mind. As a simple example, when you are looking for something, your awareness of the world around you changes. If you are looking for a new relationship, all of a sudden certain people seem to stand out in a crowd. If you are looking for a place to rest your weary feet, a curb becomes a bench.

The conscious mind has the capability to change the map. Once the map is changed, the subconscious mind, acting as the gatekeeper, begins to allow different input through the filters into consciousness. Your experience of the world will change. As a simple example of this, think about a time when you were intensely interested in something. You learned about it. You immersed yourself in it. And eventually you came to embody the new information or concept. When we embody something, it means that we have taken it into our body. It has become a part of the subconscious mind; it is imbedded into the map. After that point in time, you see things differently. Information to support your new concept pours in.

Off the Map: Breakdowns and Rebuilding

When a person encounters something of significance in their world that doesn't have a corresponding place in the internal map of reality, or when two areas of the map are found to contradict one another, the result is a breakdown. The sensation of a breakdown can be mental, physical, or emotional. Since emotions are the primary method of interface between the subconscious and the conscious minds, the sensation is normally an uncomfortable emotion. In intense people, those emotions are stronger, creating a much stronger negative emotion and a more urgent need to do something about it.

Breakdowns are the opportunities we seek in development. Every breakdown signifies that an area of the map is loosening. In some cases a part of the map actually falls apart. Growth is accomplished by allowing the parts of the map that don't serve us to fall apart and creating new areas in the map. One stumbling block for people in taking a more active mode in development is the confusion between the self and the map. If I were to believe that I am my internal map of reality, I may stubbornly refuse to change anything in my map, thinking that to do so is to deny my true self. This can only be overcome by experience, which proves otherwise. In practices 14, 15, and 16, which develop emotional intensity, we will discover the three different types of breakdowns and how to use each to the greatest advantage.

■ ■ ■

The natural state of being is to have the conscious mind and the subconscious minds working together. Both have something to offer. Each has its own strengths and purpose. Many of the practices in this book are designed to build this working relationship between the conscious and subconscious minds. The fact that these pathways between the subconscious and conscious minds are traversed by little neuropeptide molecules associated with emotion shouldn't be underestimated. If the brain is the home of the conscious mind and the body is the home of the subconscious mind, emotions are the method of communication between the two.

EVERYTHING IS RELATED TO EVERYTHING

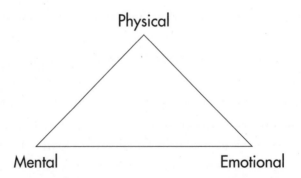

A person's experience of being includes the physical, mental, and emotional domains. They all work in concert with each other, creating our sense of self, the unique experience of being we each possess. When one of these domains changes, the other two either adapt to the change, or they act to pull the first domain back in line. Often a change in one domain causes only a temporary change. Jumping into a cool, refreshing pool will have an invigorating effect on the physical body, which will temporarily create excited thoughts and lively emotions. But these things quickly go back to the normal state. This is one of the reasons that change is so hard. We expect that we can change one domain and have it stick. For example, if you decide to go on a diet, it seems reasonable that you have only to put together a diet plan and follow it. It's logical. When it comes down to staying on the diet, the emotional and physical domains will have plenty of influence that the mental domain hadn't counted on. Feeling down, upset, or deprived in any way will easily cause a setback in the diet plan. The physical domain is capable of making a person feel tired or tense in response to dieting. Before you know it, the diet is a distant memory and the three domains are happily back in sync again.

The Physical Domain

The physical domain includes everything about your body including the subconscious mind. The way your body moves, your senses, your appetite, your breath, the way your body experiences pain and pleasure, and the physical sensations caused by psychomotor intensity are all both cause and effect in your experience of being you. But this is just the beginning. Your internal map of reality, your gatekeeper, and all the parts of your subconscious mind reside in the body. This brings new importance to the state of the physical body, the effect of sensual input, and the way you move.

The Mental Domain

The mental domain includes thoughts, reason, and just about anything going on in your conscious mind. It includes self-talk, intellectual abilities, social and cultural influences, opinions, preferences, some memories, judgments, learned skills, stories, and more. The mental domain is also both cause and effect in the total experience of being uniquely you.

The Emotional Domain

The emotional domain contains both your base mood and your emotions. The base mood is the default emotional space you live in when not influenced by a momentary emotion. Emotions are reactions to events. They aren't normally long-lived like moods. Moods and emotions are also both cause and effect in your experience while serving as a communication method between the conscious and subconscious minds.

These three domains are directly related to the five intensities; the physical domain corresponds to the sensual and psychomotor intensities, the emotional domain is the match for the emotional intensity, and the mental domain is represented by the intellectual and creative intensities. Each of the intensities is thus interrelated to the other intensities. As one type of intensity is developed, the others may be positively affected as well.

THE DRUG TO END ALL DRUGS

There's a new drug on the market. This drug has been through extensive scientific review by institutions such as Harvard,[13] Yale,[14] the National Institutes of Health,[15] Massachusetts General Hospital,[16] UCLA,[17] and other equally respectable institutions, and it has been found to have the following effects:

- A reduction in stress

- Improved cardiovascular health

- An increase in gray matter in the brain[18]

- Protective effects from recurrence of depression

- Improved attention and functioning of the prefrontal cortex

- Increased creativity

- Improved cognitive functioning

This drug has no known adverse effects. What's more, there are speculations (yet to be proven to the satisfaction of the scientific community) that this same drug may have a curative effect for addiction and provide protection against Alzheimer's disease. You haven't heard of it because no pharmaceutical company owns the patent. There's no money to be made on it because it's available to everyone at no charge. OK, it's not really new, and it's not a drug, and you may have heard of it. It's meditation. But the rest of this is true. With the advances made in brain-imaging technology, interest has been renewed in the study of meditation and its effects on the body and the mind. Meditation has been a focus of study for these institutions and others, and the benefits listed have been confirmed. But I had you going for a while, didn't I? If you could take a pill every day and get these benefits and more, would you do it?

The difference between popping a pill and meditation, and one reason many don't even try it, is that meditation takes time. It's more of an investment than popping a pill. It is also a challenge for most of us to sit still for thirty minutes or longer. It's too boring to sit and think about nothing. We crave stimulation, and underdeveloped intellectual intensity screams at the thought of thinking nothing. As difficult as it is for some to get started with meditation, I still suggest it as the most important part of this developmental journey. For our purposes, meditation has a profound effect on this process of developing intensities, particularly emotional intensity. Meditation for intense people may

- promote emotional development

- improve the witness awareness

- improve clear thinking

- reduce forgetfulness

- calm negative emotions

- clarify your personal values

- promote connection to your wiser self

- improve impulse control

My favorite benefit, and the reason I come back to meditation daily, is the inspiration. Whenever I'm feeling low, when my purpose seems distant, when my drive is lagging, meditation brings back my zest for life. Problems are put in perspective.

Athletes go through hours upon hours of physical training and practice to prepare to give their best to their sport. Actors rehearse and study lines, delivery, and movement to enable the most moving and realistic performance. Your performance in the world depends on your mind. Many of the practices in this book are based in some sort of meditative practice. They range from simple mind exercises designed to calm and soothe the body and mind to visualization exercises to sharpen the mind, to advanced contemplation. Over the years, many of us have already made up our minds about meditation. Perhaps you've heard about it or tried it and decided it just isn't for you. You may be concerned that you aren't doing it right. Or perhaps you're put off because you associate it with a religious tradition that isn't your own. Whatever your reason, I urge you to open your mind and try meditation.

Meditative practices are really just methods to improve the way your mind functions. We go through years of formal education designed to put information into our minds, but we never learn any practices to improve how our minds use the information, how to have better control over our bodies, or how to better understand and master our emotions. For intense people, meditative practices should be required coursework. They are designed to allow you to have complete command, to become a virtuoso of thought, and to master your destiny by mastering your mind. Intellectual understanding is not the same as knowing. If you miss the practices, you miss the knowing.

Even when we aren't aware of it, the noise from outside events is still running through our heads. It becomes so loud that the faint inner voice responsible for intellectual, creative, and emotional growth is drowned out. As you practice meditation, that inner voice begins to speak.

The experience of meditation varies between individuals and over time. There are times while meditating that you have a feeling that you absolutely must get up and do something right now! It is a strong feeling that should be expected. The ability to recognize it and not give in to it is built like a muscle. Each time you have that feeling during meditation, if instead of jumping up, you choose to mentally step back and watch the feeling, you are doing the equivalent of a heavy workout for that muscle. The same muscle controls impulsivity and focus.

Some people fall asleep while meditating. This is an indication that you are tired or that your struggle with a part of your internal map is overwhelming your mind. The subconscious mind may choose to do that work while you sleep. This is nothing to worry about. Just try your next meditation when you are well rested.

Sometimes there are irritating physical sensations like itches. The conscious mind will send messages similar to the "get up and go" message in order to regain control. It doesn't appreciate being asked to quiet down at first and it can put up quite a fight. This is another opportunity to work out the impulse-control muscle. You'll find that if you just accept the sensation and continue to calm your body and focus your mind, the sensation will go away. The conscious mind will need to be quiet and attentive to begin communication with the subconscious mind.

The most common experience is being distracted by thoughts. One minute you're focused, and the next you're reliving some event from yesterday or building a grocery list in your mind. When you notice this is happening, just acknowledge it and bring your mind gently back into focus. It's a good idea to check your body, as these thoughts can sometimes bring tension back into the body. Just relax your muscles again, allow your shoulders to drop back down, and breathe. Keeping the body in a relaxed state allows the subconscious mind a better avenue of communication.

After some practice, you will probably experience thoughtlessness. This is different than sleep. You are awake and aware, but there are no thoughts going through your mind, none at all. Time stands still. This experience is particularly rejuvenating. This is a time when your conscious and subconscious minds are in complete communication.

Throughout the book, many variations of meditative practice are suggested. I have heard from enough intense people that they would never be able to meditate. They have said that to sit and think of nothing is just not possible for them. Have no fear. There are several practices that involve thinking. Some even encourage a type of daydreaming. Even those who think of mediation as the ultimate form of torture should be able to find an enjoyable practice within the options presented.

THE WITNESS

The witness is a mental construct that will be your constant companion on this journey. It is an altered state of awareness, removed from your day-to-day activities, but present as they are going on. It is like watching yourself on TV or in a movie. You can see everything, feel the emotions and physical sensations, and think the thoughts while at the same time being removed from it all. The witness is not involved in the emotions or thoughts, just aware of them. It is unbiased, distanced, and at the same time, intensely interested. It is as if you are viewing your life for the first time. A part of you just watches, without judgment, as you react to the events and people in your day.

The witness is actually a higher state of awareness. The first time you experience it, you understand that the person you see, going through the automatic responses to life, can't be you, because you are watching that person. If you are able to watch it, it isn't the essence of you. Are you your arms? No, because if you lost your arms, you would still be here. Are you your voice, your senses, your thoughts, your emotions? In each case you can see that if you are able to watch these things, or if you are able to change them, they cannot be the essence of you. If they were, who would it be who is doing the watching or the changing? In many ways, the witness is the truest sense of who you are.

You may want to start by using a familiar concept like television. See yourself on a television. This television is able to share your personal unspoken thoughts and emotions as well as the picture and sound. You are watching the program of you, with great interest. You are not the one in the program, or rather, your point of view is not from inside the program. You are the viewer of the program. It goes like this as I watch the program of me:

She's been sitting at the computer for a long time now. She's turning her head to stretch her neck. It's sore. And she has a dull headache. She has an impulse to get up and go get something to eat . . . And there she goes. She's reaching for a cookie while feeling guilty at the same time. She's somehow holding the emotions of pleasure and guilt simultaneously. Interesting!

The more often you practice being in the witness state, the easier it becomes. You may even find yourself slipping into this state without trying. In the beginning it's best to give yourself a reminder. It can be something as simple as slipping a band around your wrist or wearing your watch on the other side. Each time you notice the reminder, take yourself into the witness state. This is just like building a muscle with practice and repetition.

Learning to be in a witness state can occur while you're in the midst of daily activity, if you just remember to do it. Another time to use the witness state is whenever you are upset. Any negative emotion presents a good opportunity to see an interesting show. Where is the upset in your body? How are you breathing? What thoughts are going through your head? Are your fists clenched? Does your chest hurt? Are you feeling angry, hurt, rejected, or discouraged? What story are you telling yourself about the situation? In these times you usually have to observe quickly, because the witness state doesn't allow the upset feeling to stick around for long.

The witness state allows us to observe parts of our behavior, including thoughts and emotions, from a safe-enough distance to have a better perspective. In the example, would she have noticed the connection between pleasure and guilt without the witness? This viewpoint, distanced and interested, will allow us to see the things about ourselves that are normally hidden from view. It is a glimpse into the map of the subconscious mind. We go about our days on automatic. We react to situations and encounters with people without awareness of the inner workings that provide the motivation for our actions. In order to better understand why we are the way we are, we need a different and safe perspective. The viewpoint of the witness is safe because the witness does not pass judgment. It is impartial, avoiding both justification and condemnation. It just sees what it sees. The witness will offer insights to you that were never available before. Then it is up to you to judge and decide on areas for your own personal development.

Important Points for the Impatient

- The mind is made up of the conscious mind and the subconscious mind. This model visualizes the brain as the home of the conscious mind and the body as the home of the subconscious mind. Between the two is a system of communication we call the gatekeeper, which can change the communication by altering the message or suppressing it entirely. This communication system is based on emotion.

- Within the subconscious mind is an internal map of reality used to organize the input received from the outside world. This is a smaller, condensed version of reality as we know it. This map holds all our impressions of the world, including the meanings we associate with people, places, and things.

- Most of us allow this system of input, attaching meaning and acting on it, to happen automatically throughout our lives. It is only by having our conscious minds take control that we are able to develop.

(continues)

(continued)

- Many of the methods we will use throughout this book are meditative practices that allow more open communication between the conscious and subconscious minds. Through these practices the map is revealed and we are able to take an active role in forming the map.

4

Sensual Intensity

"Bedtime"
Crooked blankets and sheets
The singular thought repeats
My feet are hot and then they're cold
Shuffling shifting uncontrolled
Hunting and searching for a comfortable spot
My feet are cold and then they're hot

The sounds of the world outside
Enter my head and collide
A rampaging battle with no clear victor
The thoughtful assault a subtle constrictor
Forcing me up as sleep retreats
To fix the crooked blankets and sheets

—STEPHAN PATTERSON

Sensual intensity is where it all begins. The senses are the only interface we have to the rest of the world. They are fundamental to how
we view the world and our everyday experience of life. With each
of the intensities, the difference is one of degree. Experiencing the

five senses with more intensity means that the world seems to hold greater pleasure and pain. This intense experience of the world is due to the gatekeeper being much more lenient. Our gatekeepers allow more to pass through. Sometimes it even seems as though they are asleep on the job.

Whether we call it "being a highly sensitive person," "sensory defensiveness," or "sensory processing sensitivity," heightened sensual sensitivity has been well recognized by psychologists. As many as 15 to 20 percent of humans are sensually intense. This ratio seems to hold true in the animal kingdom as well. In *The Highly Sensitive Person*, Dr. Elaine Aron speculates that this may be due to the advantage highly sensitive members bring to the group by being alert and aware of potential threats. She proposes that any animal species is better off having a combination of highly sensitive and not-so-sensitive members. While the highly sensitive are more aware of their surroundings, more able to discern nuances and apply greater scrutiny to their meanings, the less sensitive are more able to charge into the unknown.[19]

THE INTENSE SENSES

Sensual intensity influences the five senses, causing an increase in the effect of a stimulus. Any sight, sound, taste, touch, or smell is experienced more acutely and in more minute detail. If there were a dial controlling the input to the human system through the senses, and a "normal" person had the dial set between 1 and 5, the sensually intense person may have that dial set anywhere between 6 and 10. Along with the amplitude of the sensual input is a greater ability to discern nuances within the sensory input. The sensually intense person may notice the effects of intensity on one sense more than others.

Sensory input is not only the sights, sounds, and other purely external stimuli. The body has plenty of sensory stimulation of its own. Pain, physical discomfort, and muscle tension are sources of sensory stimulation coming from within.

Sound

Do you cover your ears when you're in a loud environment but tolerate your own music turned up high? Can you hear the minute variations between voices that make the difference between singing on key and a virtuoso performance? Have you consciously avoided places because you knew that they would be too loud? If so, you may have an expression of sensual intensity that includes sensitivity to sound. Sounds are both more irritating and more pleasant to you. The ability to hear slight variations in sound allows a greater appreciation of music. The faint sounds of wind rushing through the trees or the distant song of a bird are appreciated in depth. Unpleasant sounds are even more unpleasant. Squeaky shoes, loud motors, shrill voices, people chewing food, or the buzzing sound created by fluorescent lights cause a physical reaction very similar to pain. Even neutral sounds such as water running, children playing, or a person talking on the phone can be enough to create a level of mild tension. In tight office spaces, I've noticed that some people sitting next to a person talking more loudly than usual are able to go on with their work basically unfazed, while others can't tolerate it at all and leave the room.

Smell

Smell is said to be the strongest of senses. The route of the nerves from the nose to the brain is more direct than from the eyes or ears. It is said to be one of the older senses, predating the others, and it bypasses a relay center along the way. The route smell uses is more closely connected to the emotional parts of the brain. Interestingly enough, this is one of the senses that may be unlikely to function as well as the others due to a prevalence of allergy. Being more sensitive to the environment sometimes presents as allergic reaction. A team led by Harvard psychologist Jerome Kagan conducted a study in which the subjects, four-month-old infants, were considered "inhibited" if they showed a greater response to visual and auditory stimulation (in other words, intense). They found that 64 percent of the "inhibited" children had at least one parent with hay fever, whereas the prevalence of hay fever in the uninhibited children's parents was only 24 percent.[20] When the sense of smell is working, it, like other sensual intensities, is powerful. The smell of some foods or perfume is enough to cause nausea, while the faint scent of a loved one creates powerful emotions.

Taste

Taste is very closely related to smell. The person who was a finicky eater as a child may stay finicky, with very deliberate choices of foods that please not only by taste but also texture. There are plenty of adults who still stay away from mushrooms because of the texture, regardless of how good the taste. A refined palate may also yield a person who enjoys fine foods and has a zeal for trying new things. More common is the tendency to use food as a drug to calm the overstimulated body. Carbohydrates, cheese, and most proteins increase the level of dopamine in the system. Dopamine is the feel-good neurochemical. It has the ability to soothe away the tensions of the day. A study done at Massachusetts General Hospital showed that adults with ADHD (aka intensity) showed a 70 percent increase in dopamine transporters.[21] That means that there is less free dopamine in the system. The study was not able to determine whether the increase in dopamine transmitters was cause or effect, meaning the increase could be due to the brain searching out dopamine, or it could be that the increased transporters were the cause. Of course, smoking, alcohol, and macaroni and cheese are natural dopamine generators, so we are extremely tempted by them and other drugs.

Sight

With sight, the senses can be both bombarded and fine-tuned. A sensitivity to light, particularly bright or flashing lights, is a sign of sensual intensity. Some days the sun is too bright. The sense of sight can also be bombarded by too many things to see. Did you ever walk into a store and feel overwhelmed, the shelves filled with such variety that it actually made you tired? The only reason my cluttered house doesn't wear me out is that I've stopped seeing most of it. Sometimes I move treasured items around just so that I can notice them again. My nonintense husband accuses me of moving things just to bother him. He likes a place for everything and everything in its place. Really that has nothing to do with it. The real delights in sensual intensity of the visual kind are artistic expression and appreciation. Beauty can be found everywhere. A curled and fallen leaf is a masterpiece. The dirt on a city street makes a mosaic. The veins and wrinkles in an aging hand, colors splashed against a drop cloth for painting, or the angelic face of a sleeping child are unexpected and constant reminders of the gift of this particular intensity.

Touch

Every move we make through the world requires touching pieces of it. All day, every day, we are feeling the sensations of clothing. Every relationship involves some level of touch from the very professional handshake to the intimate embrace. Even when we are sleeping, we are being touched by our bedding. This particular sense, when experienced intensely, is inescapable. Tags in clothing can be irritating. Seams in socks, wool sweaters, hats or headbands, and tight waistbands can be unbearable. Even the air around us can be a source of irritation if it's too hot, too cold, or contains any allergens. Goldilocks was definitely intense. As she tried every bed in the home of the three bears, she found one too soft, one too hard, and one just right. It's like that with us. A massage can easily be too hard, but if it's too light, so as to tickle, it's just as bad. We have to find the "just right" feeling of everything that touches us.

Inner Touch

The senses aren't limited to the ones with which we experience the outside world. Our internal experience of bodily sensations is another sense. Nerves are everywhere in our bodies and they all send sensory input to the brain. The nervous system controlling the inner workings of the body is there to tell us when something is wrong, so most of the inner sensations we notice are unpleasant. A stomach ache is felt just as intensely as anything else. With internal sensory input it's much harder to recognize the differences between "normal" and intense experience. Aches and pains, digestion, heartburn, or a nervous stomach may seem to be experienced by all with the same intensity, but we know that isn't true. One of my sons was able to feel an ear infection coming on almost before the doctor could see it. I remember the doctor telling me that while yes, he does have a slight ear infection, he shouldn't be able to feel anything yet. The nervous system within the body is also capable of experiencing pleasure. The satisfaction of a full stomach, the energy that wells up from excitement, and the pleasure of movement are all examples.

HOW SENSUAL INTENSITY
AFFECTS US

In the jungle of a human city, sensual intensity is a challenge. Since most of the developed world is created with less sensitivity in mind, the average level of stimulation is too much for the sensitive individual. The way we take in sensory information differs from others in that our gatekeepers allow much more to get through. Or perhaps we are perceiving things normally, and it's the majority of people who have some level of sensory deprivation. Regardless of which stance you take, we do experience sensory input differently. We not only seem to amplify the input, but also process it differently. It's as if the sensual input is dissected into smaller parts. We notice nuances, so for every external stimulus there is more information to process. While this may explain how we are sometimes able to learn without realizing we are learning, it also uses more energy.

The world is much more uncomfortable and at times hostile for us than it is for nonintense people. Societies would never create lights too bright or sound levels so high that the average person would be in pain when exposed to them. In the few situations where this is inevitable, like working on an airport runway, protective gear is required. The sensually intense person, however, encounters too much sensory arousal on a daily basis. A constant, even if minor, amount of too much sensory stimulation causes a person to tense against the discomfort or attempt to avoid it altogether. Bracing oneself occurs primarily on an unconscious level, so that at the end of a day it isn't obvious as the source of exhaustion. To test this theory, see how a one-hour walk in the forest or on the beach compares with a one-hour walk through a crowded shopping mall. If it were the walking that caused a person to feel tired, the result would be the same. For most sensually intense people, this little exercise doesn't even need to be played out. You already know how much more tiring the hour spent in a crowded area with too much going on would affect you. The effect of sensory overload impacts more than energy levels. Remember that everything is related to everything. Sensory overload can have a profound impact on moods and emotions, making one more prone to grumpiness. It can also overwhelm the mind, creating confusion or a foggy thought sensation.

Perhaps the most interesting effect of sensual intensity is on the way we process information. First, we take information in with more detail. Every one of our senses is so highly tuned that small variations that a more "normal" person might generalize away are part of our normal perceptions. While the "normal" person may generalize a person upon first meeting as, say, a middle-aged man with graying hair and a mustache, the sensually intense person takes in the entire essence of the person. There is a feel to him, a manner, and a certain presence. These perceptions are the result of subtle details in the way he talks or moves. He has an emotional aura unique to him. He also has a sound and perhaps a smell. These things are all taken in. The impression of the person becomes a more complex gestalt. When some part of the outward appearance of that person changes, it may not even be noticed by the sensually intense person if the change hasn't impacted the overall impression. He could shave his mustache, which would be a big change to a more sensually normal person, and it may not be noticed by the sensually intense person. On the other hand, the sensually intense person would definitely notice if his demeanor had changed.

We also take in more information because it is paired with sensual intensity. We talked about the gatekeeper in chapter 3. The gatekeeper has three criteria for allowing information into the mind. The input must either present a threat, be of interest, or be something the conscious mind has instructed the gatekeeper to look for. When information comes in with a strong emotion, or with pain, it is interpreted by the gatekeeper as a threat. Everything surrounding an experience associated with pain goes straight past the gatekeeper. He doesn't even stop them to ask for credentials. Since the sensually intense person experiences so much more physical discomfort on a daily basis, there's a lot of information gliding right past that gatekeeper. More information means a more complex inner experience. It's not just pain from lights that are too bright or sounds that are too loud. All the intensities contribute to the overload, which creates this pass through the doors of the gatekeeper.

Dr. Elaine Aron explains this overload as overarousal. She contends that there is an optimal level of arousal that everyone seeks. The sensually intense person, which she describes as highly sensitive, has more difficulty achieving optimal arousal since we are more easily aroused. In *The Highly Sensitive Person*, Dr. Aron compares the body to an infant. Just as we would care for an infant by keeping them fed when they are hungry, warm and protected from the cold, and entertained just enough but not too much, we should also care for our physical selves. In an attempt to self-regulate our level of arousal, whether conscious or unconscious, we may turn to substances and activities that dial it back by increasing certain neurochemicals, primarily dopamine. Alcohol, food, and many drugs all dial down the intensity by providing more dopamine.

Dialing back the intensity isn't always desirable. Sensual intensity gives us the ability to appreciate life in the way of an artist. Dr. Dabrowski noted that sensual intensity is quite often paired with creative intensity, and it's no wonder. A person who can deeply appreciate the beauty of nature or hear a symphony in the song of a bird is that much more likely to be driven to creativity. Each of our senses is designed to create both pleasure and pain. We're well aware of the pain, but have we fully experienced the pleasure? When was the last time you did something great for your body just to enjoy the feeling? When did you last enjoy a warm bath by candlelight or stand completely still on the beach at sunset, just to feel the ocean breeze kiss your skin? Do you remember when you last came in from the cold and warmed your hands by a fire? Can you close your eyes and remember the delectable aromas and sounds coming from the kitchen while a meal is being prepared? All these things and more are like gifts if you choose to slow down enough to savor them. You can choose to accept one of these gifts any time you like. Sensual intensity makes these moments every day.

In order to fully appreciate and develop sensual intensity I propose taking a stand to refuse to dial it back. The pleasures are too wonderful to miss, so the solution has to be to reduce the pain and keep all the pleasure.

Important Points for the Impatient

- Our senses are our only interface with the world. Being sensually intense means that our experience of the world is more intense.

- We are more sensitive to pain, making the world seem a harsh place at times. This is balanced by being more attuned to the beauty around us.

- The natural way our brains store information takes advantage of sensual intensity making us much more complex.

5

Sensual Practices: Make Me Safe and Warm

The fear response is deeply ingrained in the human brain. Under threat of any kind—hunger, thirst, pain, shame, confusion, or too much, too new or too fast—we respond in ways to keep us safe. Our minds will focus only on the information that is, at that moment, important for survival. Fear kills curiosity and inhibits exploration.

—BRUCE D. PERRY, MD, PHD, "CREATING AN
EMOTIONALLY SAFE CLASSROOM"

Development of sensual intensity is destined to be a rewarding undertaking. What could be better than to remove sources of pain and find in their place a safe and secure world offering the most wonderful, sensual pleasures? The sensually intense person has already endured plenty of pain and discomfort in this life, regardless of their age. The difficulties can be put aside and life can start anew with the two practices outlined herein. Please take your time with these, experience them fully and get as much as possible out of each step. Your quality of life depends on it.

Practice 1

PROTECTING YOUR SENSUALLY INTENSE SELF

Sensitive people experience more pain than most. Because of this you have learned to brace yourself. From the time you were a baby, you have experienced pain caused by what should have been normal stimuli in the environment. Everything from the light of the sun to hugs and kisses from well-meaning relatives may have caused some discomfort. As adults the pain continues. Graphic images on TV, the stench of exhaust fumes, fluorescent lighting, office temperatures that are too hot or too cold, or sitting for too long in traffic can all cause enough discomfort to make you tense against the pain to come, real or anticipated. The remainder of your ability to grow with this program depends on starting from a place where you know you are safe and protected.

There may be a history of denying your sensitivity, particularly for men. You may have developed stories to explain yourself to others that avoid the very real physical differences you experience. Have you heard yourself say that you just don't care for massages? Do you make excuses to miss events like a trip to Las Vegas or some other place that bombards your senses? It's almost as if anything is better than the truth. Well, it's time to stop. And with the end of the excuses comes the end of the idea that you just need to toughen up. You've tried that and you're living the result. You can appear "normal" and try to push the pain from your consciousness. However the pain doesn't stay pushed. It manifests in some way every time. There is no need to pretend that you aren't sensitive or to apologize for it. Claim your sensitivity. This is a bold move that sets the tone for the remainder of the steps in this book. It is time to accept and cherish your way of sensing the world.

For those closest to you there is a need to educate them on your sensual sensitivity. There is plenty of literature for them to read. They can Google "highly sensitive people" or "sensory processing sensitivity." This is very real and not as uncommon as one might believe.[22]

To recognize the onset of overwhelm, it will help to go back to the witness we created previously. Step into the position of the witness as soon as you recognize overwhelm. Watching yourself go into sensory overwhelm only a few times will provide a solid foundation so that you can begin to recognize the signs and the situations.

When you better understand the situations and environments that produce overwhelm for you, begin to plan. If a long exposure to crowds is going to burn as surely as a long exposure to the sun, you can design your interactions by limiting time you spend in crowds or by creating intermissions where you can be alone. If a schedule that demands you rush every morning ensures that you start every day overwhelmed, you can change your schedule.

Make a list of the changes you can make to protect yourself. Here are some suggestions that may help you to get started. This will be an ongoing process. As you eliminate the top one or two, you may find that another source of discomfort comes to your attention as a cause of pain. Keep going until your days aren't filled with pain anymore.

- Say no to invitations that will place you in an environment that is too loud or too busy.

- Plan recuperation time following busy events. This can be a planned "spa day" after a busy holiday or just a nap after a trying morning at the DMV.

- Create a routine to end your day that relaxes your body and mind before bed such as a warm bath or reading an inspirational book with a cup of chamomile tea.

- Add an exercise routine to your day to relax the nervous system.

- Get rid of clothes that aren't comfortable. Life's too short!

- Lighting counts! Replace bright lights with lower-wattage bulbs. Lamps are much easier on the eyes than overhead lighting. Definitely cover any exposed light bulbs and avoid fluorescent lights.

- Replace your bedding with the best you can afford. I found that bamboo sheets are smoother than silk, breathe as well as cotton, and are more durable.

- Spend fifteen minutes when you get home from work with a heating pad on any tense muscles.

- Use fabric softener in your laundry.

- Use sound-blocking headphones when in loud places like an airplane or subway.

- Take mini muscle relaxation breaks during the day. In your mind go from the tips of your toes to the top of your head tensing and then relaxing each muscle group.

- Finally, it is well worth having a slightly uncomfortable conversation to teach your mate how to touch you. It may be the first time they understand why you are the way you are. This is a completely loving act that can only help to ensure the future success of the relationship.

Moving from planning into the changes your system requires to be whole and healthy is a big step for some. If you are accustomed to adjusting, to taking care of others, or to sucking it up, the steps you've planned may feel selfish. This is where you have to leave your usual ways behind and give something new a try. If you can't do something differently than you have been doing, you're stuck. The idea is to move from changes occurring without your input or control to changes occurring because you designed them and brought them into being. This is where the rubber meets the road. Drive.

Practice 2

CREATING A SAFE AND HOSPITABLE WORLD

As long as the subconscious mind stays the same, the world stays the same. It sounds ridiculous because, of course, your subconscious mind doesn't control the world, but it does control your perception of the world through your internal map of reality. The subconscious doesn't make decisions. It doesn't plan. Like the Internet, it accepts any information that is fed to it regardless of quality, and it spits it back regardless of quality.

The conscious mind is the only part of the mind that can evaluate the quality of information and make decisions. While in the passive mode, the conscious mind doesn't get to exercise any power over the contents of the map. In the active mode, the conscious mind is in complete control. We will need to design the message we want to introduce to the subconscious mind and then deliver it. The subconscious takes in information from the conscious mind in the form of a thought/emotion package and by using repetition. The best method is to combine these two avenues into what can be referred to as intense concentration. We're going to use that information to remove the information from the subconscious mind that isn't useful or in support of our goals and to replace it with information that will better support us.

PREPARE A MESSAGE FOR THE SUBCONSCIOUS

Let's design the information we want to feed to the subconscious mind. In order to progress through this program and to fulfill the promise of this book, you will need to start from a place of safety. If that requirement isn't met, the rest of the program will be weaker and may not produce the result you want. Because of the effect of sensual intensity on your view of the world, the first message to the subconscious should begin to counteract the expectation of danger and pain.

There are a few requirements for crafting the actual message, and one of them is *not* that the message is true. Remember, you are currently determining true and false based on your current internal map of reality. If the message sounds true to you, and it matches the results you're getting in life, there's no need to plant it in the subconscious. It's already there. The message you need to plant will probably sound untrue and even dangerous. How does this message cause your conscious mind to react? "I am completely safe in the world," or "The world is an entirely safe place." Most likely there are some immediate and emphatic responses about how dangerous it would be to believe that.

The information we need to store in the subconscious mind should be formed based on how useful that information will be to our cause, not on whether or not it currently sounds true. It can be tested against people who seem to have already accomplished what we want to accomplish, or who have the approach to life we would like to have. What do they believe? Do they believe that the world is a dangerous place? Probably not.

The message should be stated in the present tense because the present is all that the subconscious mind understands. So a statement like "The world will be safe for me" is not helpful. It has to be in present tense such as "The world is safe for me," or "I walk safely through the world."

The message also must be in positive terms. The subconscious mind doesn't process negatives well and will turn them into positives. So a statement like "There is no danger in the world" gets translated into "Danger in the world." A good test is to take each word separately and see what kind of message it would send. If any word in the message you're constructing has a negative meaning, change it.

SENDING THE MESSAGE

In order to put the conscious and subconscious mind in the best communication, we have to enter a different brain wave pattern. This conscious move to a different brain wave pattern is accomplished after much meditation practice. The methods vary but the concept is the same: Quiet the body and slow down the mind. The problem that intense people have with this is that it's pretty boring. We have more to quiet than most and the chatter and activity in our minds is a constant companion. The conscious mind basically throws a temper tantrum whenever we try to have it sit quietly.

I have two solutions for this. The first is to cheat using a meditation aid. The one I use is based on binaural beat technology. By feeding different frequencies into each ear, the brain resolves the differences by entering into a slower frequency. This allows the meditation CD to take your brain easily from a waking state to a deep state of meditation without any effort on your part. I use Bill Harris's Holosync system, which is available at *www.centerpointe.com*.

The second solution is to skip the meaningless mantra used by most meditators and jump straight to the message you want to introduce to your subconscious mind. Your conscious mind will still complain, but you'll have something to offer it when it does.

This is a daily practice best done at the same time of day and in the same place.

1. Start by selecting a quiet and comfortable place to sit. Set a timer that will gently remind you when your time is up. After a while you'll find that you can easily go over thirty minutes. Start with only fifteen minutes and stretch it to thirty minutes after about two weeks. Some people like to go longer. It's really a personal choice, but thirty minutes is enough. Depending upon your schedule, going longer than an allotted time may be a problem. If it is, take steps to remove the concern from your mind. (A caution here: Any alarm is going to be louder and more startling when you are meditating. Choose one that is very gentle and quiet. There are soft chimes and other types of alarms available under the category of meditation alarms or chimes. If you are using the meditation CD from Centerpointe, the sound will change after thirty minutes, so no alarm is needed.)

2. Prepare the body. This should be done while seated upright without any back support if possible. The spine being straight and the muscles being relaxed is important to allow the subconscious to function well. Use the half-lotus position if it's comfortable for you (legs crossed). Sit still with your eyes closed. Now relax your muscles. In the beginning you may need to go from toes to head or head to toes tensing and relaxing each muscle group. This can be done with each breath. Breathe in and tense your feet and toes. Breathe out and relax them. Repeat the same thing with the next breath with the legs, then the torso, arms, neck, then head and face, until your body feels more relaxed. After you've practiced this for a while, you'll be able to relax your muscles very quickly

without going through this step by step. Now your subconscious mind is ready to communicate.

3. Quiet your mind. The chatter that normally goes on in the conscious mind makes it very hard to have any communication outside the conscious mind. In order to communicate with the subconscious mind, the conscious mind has to learn to be quiet. Start by repeating your message to the subconscious. Say it slowly in your mind. Keep repeating it in your mind. Your thoughts will wander. That's natural even for experienced meditators. Don't let it bother you. Just watch as if from a distance, like an impartial observer. When you realize that you've wandered off, go back to your message. You can beef up the message and keep yourself more engaged by imagining situations where you feel safe. Vividly imagine the scene and feel the feeling of safety. Keep doing this until the time is up. When the time is up, come back to the world slowly. Give your conscious and subconscious a few minutes to part instead of tearing them away from each other.

This practice is only the beginning. It can be thought of as your formal introduction to your subconscious mind. After a few days or weeks of asking your conscious mind to tell your subconscious mind that the world is safe, the gatekeeper will start producing evidence to support it. This method will allow you to absolutely transform your world by transforming the information your subconscious mind and the gatekeeper allow into your conscious mind. If this has you all tingly with excitement at the possibilities this holds, you're on the right track.

Important Points for the Impatient

- Practice 1: Protecting Your Sensually Intense Self reduces the chance of painful experiences by increasing your control over your environment. In this step, sensory overload is reduced, the physical environment is modified to be less invasive, and we finally claim our sensual intensity. This step marks the end of "toughening up" or making excuses.

- Practice 2: Creating a Safe and Hospitable World reprograms your subconscious mind so that a new, safer, and more hospitable world is created for you. This safer world allows you to appreciate the benefits of sensual intensity without the threats.

6

Psychomotor Intensity

Life should not be a journey to the grave with the intention of arriving safely in a pretty and well preserved body, but rather to skid in broadside in a cloud of smoke, thoroughly used up, totally worn out, and loudly proclaiming "Wow! What a Ride!"
—HUNTER S. THOMPSON

Have you ever had a sudden urge to say or do something that seemed to overtake you? An urge is an involuntary, natural, or instinctive impulse.[23] Compare an urge to the feeling you get when you have to go to the bathroom. It's not something that can be put off for long. The longer you try, the more intense the feeling becomes. You begin to feel physically uncomfortable until finally there is no choice. Better judgment becomes fuzzy. That gas station restroom that would have been unthinkable to use an hour ago starts to look like just the right solution to the problem.

Psychomotor intensity is an urge to act. The brain tells the body to move into action, and it has almost no choice. It feels just as uncontrollable as any other physical urge. The only choice is to act on it in some way, or suffer the consequences. The term "psychomotor" refers to movement of the body as it relates to mental activity. This has everything to do with the nervous system. The motor cortex of the brain is as susceptible to increased activity as any other portion of the brain. When this area of the brain is stimulated, it sends messages to the body to move. As with all the intensities, psychomotor intensity is a matter of degree. The outward expression can appear to be hyperactivity, although in adults it is often pushed underground. There may be a tendency to expel physical energy by talking, tapping or wiggling some body part, or excessive hand movements.

Because of the amount of stimulation to the motor cortex, the intense person is endowed with a greater-than-average compulsion to take action. It can be expressed in different ways, both negative and positive. The trick is to understand how you have been dealing with this difference and learn to allow your natural tendency toward taking action to be both easily managed and a benefit in accomplishing things.

YOU ARE AN OPEN ENERGY SYSTEM

With any living system, including human beings, as energy goes in, energy must go out. It's a natural cycle or rhythm. Systems theory has been used to understand everything from biological systems to mathematics. The basis is that living systems are not stand-alone things. They interact with their environment, and the environment interacts with them, changing both. An open system takes in and releases energy, information, and materials. The input to the system may fluctuate at times. The system needs to be somewhat flexible in order to expand and contract with the fluctuations in the current input and ability to output. For example, as you feed food into your stomach, it is able to expand. If less food goes in, it contracts. The same flexibility exists throughout the human system, but the system has limits. When pushed beyond that limit, the system begins to behave in unexpected ways or break down.

The food we take in, the sensory input, and the interaction with other people are all forms of energy, information, and materials going into the system. Activity and expression of thoughts, ideas, and emotions are all energy going out of the system. Most people have a natural flow of energy going in and out that allows the "system" to remain at a relatively constant state. The natural expression of energy is within socially accepted norms. Intense people have an energy intensifier. This creates a situation where the amount of energy going into the system is intensified, resulting in a need for the amount of energy going out to increase in order to maintain balance in the system.

If the natural expression of this energy is deemed to be socially unacceptable, a person may try to hold more energy in or express it in secreted ways. Please pardon the return to bathroom talk, but this is a great example. If your body needs to expel gas, and farting is considered unacceptable—which it is, guys—then you may try holding it in, letting it out slowly, or sneaking off into an empty corridor to let it all out. If you hold it in, it's just going to cause pain and it will eventually have to come out anyway. If you try to let out a slow one, it may turn into a squeaker . . . uh oh. Or if you find an empty corridor to let it all fly, you have either isolated yourself or run the risk of having been found out.

So it is with psychomotor intensity. It has to come out. Those who let it fly run a risk of being considered socially unacceptable. Those who try to hold it in suffer emotional pain that may manifest as agitation, aggression, anxiety, or anger. The stress associated with blocked energy creates not only emotional suffering but also disease. Those who try to hide it may get caught in a cycle of substance abuse, overeating, nervous habits, risk-taking behaviors, or working compulsively.

PSYCHOMOTOR EFFECTS ON THE PHYSICAL DOMAIN

The physical experience of psychomotor intensity includes both joy in the physical expression of energy and discomfort in the form of tension associated with stopping the flow.

Joy in Fast or Urgent Action—Spurt Work

Physical expression of psychomotor intensity is the most natural form of release. When the body is being told by the central nervous system to get into action, action feels good. As adults we don't always take heed of these messages sent by the brain. Running around, jumping, flailing of arms, and skipping are all too juvenile. We do have adult ways of expending energy, but we tend to make those all business and no fun. Working out, running, housework, and the like will accomplish the same purpose, but they are not nearly as much fun as the unbridled exuberance that we were allowed to express as children. But that doesn't have to mean that we have no outlet for energy.

Our energy likes to come out in spurts. I have no idea why this is; it's just something I've noticed in all the intense people I know and have coached. Long, sustained releases of energy like long-distance running are not as satisfying as sprints. We so enjoy the urgency and the release that we'll actually use it to get things done. Waiting until the last minute to clean before company arrives is much more fun than having regular daily chores to ensure that the house is always clean. Creating a sense of urgency by waiting until the last minute seems to make the job enjoyable for spurt workers. It also removes all doubt that it has to be done. "It's now or never" is a great motivator. If there is a larger job to do, breaking it up into smaller jobs and taking a break in between seems to work better. Understanding this natural pattern of energy release can help in selecting a workout routine or a method of accomplishing almost anything. If your energy is best in spurts, plan to work in spurts. There is no reason we have to expend energy the same slow and steady way as our less intense friends.

Just as I have used this to help intense children get their homework done, you can use this to get almost anything done. Create urgency and work in spurts. The really wonderful part of this method, aside from being able to get things done, is that it does a great job of releasing psychomotor energy.

Vocalization

The motor cortex, the area of the brain that controls our voluntary motor functions, allocates about a third of its space to vocalization and anything associated with the mouth. The act of talking serves to release psychomotor energy every bit as much as running. Just as psychomotor intensity that manifests in the large muscles is a cause for misdiagnosis of boys as having ADHD, the manifestation of the very same energy in the form of talking is completely missed in many girls. Although I believe 100 percent of the ADHD diagnoses to be misdiagnoses, I think the reason that boys are diagnosed more than twice as often as girls is that girls are more likely to express "hyperactivity" vocally.

Busy Hands

Another third of the motor cortex is devoted to the hands. The release of excess energy through the hands can be seen in the gesture of hand wringing. Often mistaken to mean distress, it is really a relief of physical tension for many people. Many intense people have habits of drumming their fingers or using their hands in gestures while talking. Nail biting and picking at scabs are also signs of motor intensity. Crafts and other activities that keep the hands moving are therapeutic.

Restlessness

Energy that is not released creates tension in the body. Thomas Edison said, "Restlessness is discontent, and discontent is the first necessity of progress. Show me a thoroughly satisfied man, and I will show you a failure." This is another benefit of this intensity. If we want to build energy for something, we have a ready supply. If that energy is not expressed physically or vocally, it will begin to grow as restlessness. That restlessness brings the emotional and mental domains with it. We will have no choice but to create emotions and thoughts in harmony with restlessness. This combination can create the motivation for change, be it positive or negative. Restlessness motivates precisely because it's uncomfortable.

Sleeplessness

Psychomotor intensity can cause sleep disturbances. It keeps the brain activity level so high that relaxing into sleep is difficult. This may be noticed in babies that never seem to sleep; however, this isn't an intensity that we outgrow. It stays with us, and we forget to connect the childhood behaviors with the adult behaviors. A fussy and colicky baby will very likely grow into an adult with psychomotor intensity.

Muscle Tension—Aches and Pains

A side effect of holding in physical energy is muscle pain. The area from the shoulders to the top of the head is referred to as the tension triangle. The muscles in this triangle are the most likely to suffer from holding in energy. It may manifest as headaches, upper back pain, forehead tension, or teeth grinding.

PSYCHOMOTOR EFFECTS ON THE EMOTIONAL DOMAIN

Psychomotor intensity is a strong physical influence, and as such, it has a lasting impact on our thoughts and feelings. So constant is this impact that we don't normally realize its origin. It has been with us and creating a certain genre of thought and a unique force on our emotions since birth. Some common emotional consequences of psychomotor intensity are ambition, frustration, anger, and resentment.

Ambition

The urge to take action, if not subdued by artificial means, is a form of ambition. This is not ambition as in the desire for honor or fame. This type of ambition is the pure desire and sometimes need to take action. This ambition carries with it a positive relationship with possibility. A life view that includes the belief that it's possible to bring about improvements in the future by taking action predisposes a person to a certain type of mood about life. Ambition by itself is neither good nor bad. The result of an action taken can be good or bad, effective to bring about the desired change, or ineffective.

Frustration

Frustration is the emotion created when an effort, attempt, or desire is thwarted. Imagine running as fast as you can, putting everything into it, only to discover that some giant has been holding on to your belt from behind, ensuring that you can make no progress. You pull yourself away and try again when you realize that someone has greased the track. Despite all your efforts, you can't gain any traction, and again you make no progress. That's frustration, and it is a natural shadow side to ambition. When you have true ambition and it either can't be acted on or the actions don't produce the desired result, frustration is a natural response.

Anger and Resentment

When the ambition/frustration package is combined with resentment, anger and possibly aggression ensue. Resentment is the assessment of things not being as they should be. Idealists, as we are inclined to be, have an easy time pronouncing things to be other than ideal. Since an ideal is by definition a model of perfection, and since perfection either exists everywhere or nowhere—depending on your perspective—the idealist has easy pickings. Any domain of life, any person or situation, can be fodder for focusing on what is not as it should be. An imperfection in another person, particularly if the imperfection is judged to be the cause of some injury or insult, provides the starting point for the cycle of anger, which goes like this: *That shouldn't have happened. He not only hurt me (or someone else) but also could have done otherwise. That person (or system, or organization, etc.) is to blame and should be punished.*

The difference between resentment and anger is in the expression. Resentment is private, held internally. Anger is the outward expression. It is more public. When a person is in the mood of resentment and is also predisposed to taking action, anger is a likely result. In these cases traditional anger management training doesn't work very well because it doesn't address the underlying cause of the troubled emotions. In general, traditional therapies are ill informed on intensity.

PSYCHOMOTOR EFFECTS ON THE MENTAL DOMAIN

Each thought accompanied by psychomotor intensity carries with it a sense of importance. Muscle tension and heightened nerves create a sense of urgency. We then confuse urgency with importance. The result is that most thoughts seem to be important. We think that our thoughts are so important that we can't choose to release them. Competing thoughts, neither of which can be discarded, can cause long-term internal conflict. A client of mine summed it up saying that abandoning her thought would be like throwing away a child. Even thoughts that aren't productive, which provide no possibility and produce only internal tension, are deemed too important to release.

Although all types of thoughts are influenced by psychomotor intensity, certain genres of thought are more common due to the combination of intense energy and the accompanying emotional field. In a process called the "linguistic reconstruction of emotions," any emotion can be reconstructed through language to determine the essential thought elements of that emotion. It's not required that the thoughts precede the emotion. Because the three elements of physical, emotional, and mental must be in balance, the emotion can and often does create the thought. We are meaning-making machines.

Thoughts associated with a particular emotion may vary slightly from individual to individual, but the basic pattern remains the same. Because we know the emotions common to psychomotor intensity, we have an insight to the thoughts that would accompany them. The emotions of ambition, frustration, and anger all have roots in an assessment that things are not as they should be. These emotions give rise to thoughts. Remember, the thought doesn't always precede the emotion.

Thoughts That Accompany Ambition

To find the linguistic reconstruction of any emotion, we start with an assertion. An assertion is a fact, something that cannot be disputed and is not a matter of opinion. "I assert that X has happened" is a pretty safe first step for the reconstruction of any emotion since emotions are typically based on a reaction to something. After the assertion there are one or more assessments that are nothing more than judgments made about the event that has happened provided by the internal map of reality. With ambition there is an assessment that there is something to be done about a situation or event. Another assessment required for ambition is the self-assessment of being prepared and capable of doing that something. Finally, most emotional reconstructions conclude with a declaration of what is to follow. A declaration is a statement that creates something, such as an intention to do something. A great example of a declaration is the Declaration of Independence. A declaration is so because I say it is so.

For ambition, the declaration would be about taking action. When we put it all together, it looks like this:

"I assert that X has happened (or I would like X to happen)."

"I assess that something needs to be done about X."

"I assess myself to be prepared and capable of doing something about X."

"I declare my intention to take action."

The linguistic reconstruction of emotions allows us to predict the thoughts that would be expected to go with the combined emotional field of ambition and intense physical energy. They would have to be in alignment with the assessments of something needing to happen and thoughts of being able and prepared to take some action.

Thoughts That Accompany Frustration

Frustration is very closely related to ambition in that they are both born of a desire to accomplish something. When something gets in the way of that accomplishment or of taking action, the result is frustration. A declaration of frustration might look like this:

"I assert that X happened (or didn't happen)."

"I assess that I intended or wanted something to occur."

"I assess that something is thwarting that as a possibility for me."

"I declare my predisposition to cry out, complain, or take any action available."

Thoughts created in frustration are about finding a more forceful way forward, giving up in a huff, or crying out for help. When a person is frustrated and experiencing psychomotor intensity, thoughts of action predominate, but they differ from the thoughts related to ambition in that they are permissive of more drastic action.

Thoughts That Accompany Anger

Frustration and anger both produce thoughts about what is wrong. Both may also create thoughts of how someone (or something) is not doing what he should be doing. The biggest difference is that frustration is usually turned inward, while anger is turned outward. A declaration of anger might be one of the following:

"I assert that X happened."

"I assess that X caused some damage to me."

"I assess that someone is responsible for that."

"I assess that that person could have done otherwise."

"I declare a predisposition to punish that person."

BEING IN THE FLOW

Psychomotor intensity has both positive and negative aspects. The point of this chapter is to awaken awareness of both. In the development of psychomotor intensity, the goal is to eliminate physical suffering and create a smooth, healthy flow of energy. Understanding your nature, and the futility of trying to go against your nature, provides a foundation. The next steps are designed to bring relief from the potential suffering and develop awareness of the inherent power of this intensity. Only by being aware of our power and using it effectively can we be masters of our energy.

I've often compared intense people to race cars. You're either on or off. If you're on, you're going. The slow and steady pace of an economy car would kill your engine. This is your nature. The most important thing is for you to understand and embrace your nature. In order to do that with psychomotor intensity, you have to be aware of your ideal flow of energy. Clearing out the clogs in the engine, then running it so that clogs don't occur again puts you in a very powerful position.

Important Points for the Impatient

- Psychomotor intensity is created by the motor cortex in the brain. The motor cortex is divided roughly into three sections. One section controls the large muscles, another controls the mouth and vocalization, and the last third controls the hands.

- You are an open system. Energy goes in and energy flows out. A balance must be maintained in order for the system to survive. Intensity causes the inbound energy to be amplified, which in turn causes the need to release more energy than the average person.

- When the expression of psychomotor intensity is blocked, the flow is interrupted, and tension is the result. This blocked energy creates restlessness, sleeplessness, and muscle tension.

- Understanding your nature, and the futility of trying to go against your nature, provides a foundation for creating a smooth flow of psychomotor energy. In order to do that with psychomotor intensity, you have to be aware of the ideal flow of energy for you. Clearing out the clogs in the engine, and then running it so that clogs don't occur again, puts you in a very powerful position.

7

Psychomotor Practices:
It's My Energy, Dammit!

The first idea that the child must acquire, in order to be actively disciplined, is that of the difference between good and evil; and the task of the educator lies in seeing that the child does not confound good with immobility and evil with activity.

—MARIA MONTESSORI

Ultimately, psychomotor intensity provides both energy to accomplish things and radiant energy in the form of charisma or magnetism. When the intense energy that flows through your body travels without interruption, when it is smooth and natural, when it is accompanied by thoughts and emotions of courage, confidence, and power, people will notice your energy when you walk into a room. When it is tempered with kindness and openness, people are drawn to you. You become a magnet.

The importance of having clear energy and information pathways is evident when we see that those energy pathways impact our physical and emotional health. In these exercises I've included a way to clear out energy blocks held in your body, a demonstration of how the way you move opens or closes ways of being for you, and an awareness of how to select a regular exercise routine that not only releases energy but expands your capacity for being in different dispositions than your norm. My intention in these exercises is not to reduce the amount of energy flowing through you, but rather to help you clear the channels, tune the energy, and enjoy the flow.

Don't hide your energy anymore. Be proud. Let it flow freely through you and gain access to one of the best kept secrets of intensity, the power to act.

Practice 3

WALK A MILE IN MY SHOES

The way you move your body has an impact on your emotional self and the thoughts you entertain. It actually has a fundamental impact on your outlook. This fun exercise proves the point. This is best done if you have a willing participant, lest you be thought a stalker, but I've done this while walking behind someone in a shopping center without being noticed.

1. Ask your participant to walk normally around in a circle or down a street for at least five minutes. Walk behind them and mimic their movements. Watch closely for the way the head moves and the angle of the gaze. Notice how much the arms sway and the position of the hands. How far off the ground does each foot come up, and what part of the foot meets the ground first on the down step? Is the pace fast or slow? Do the hips sway, or are they steady? How is the chest held? After you're satisfied that you are mimicking their movements exactly, keep walking and feel the movements.

2. Now check in with yourself. How are you feeling (and feeling foolish doesn't count)? Do you feel strong or weak, tired or invigorated, sexy, determined, hurried or worried? Ask yourself what your outlook is on life at this very moment as you walk.

3. When you think you've got it, share your findings with your friend. In almost every case this will turn out to be a little spooky to your friend. They will not understand how you were able to gain the insights about them that you did.

This is what is meant by "walk a mile in my shoes." It can show you what it feels like to be that person. By imitating the way a person moves, you will begin to feel the feelings they are feeling and think the thoughts they are thinking. The point is, the way you move is not innocent. It has a direct and profound impact on your mood, your outlook on life, and the types of thoughts you can think.

Practice 4

BEING STILL AND CREATING FLOW

A natural side effect of psychomotor intensity, particularly if it isn't fully expressed, is muscle tension. In order to progress on the path laid out in this book, the first step is to learn to relax your muscles at will. This is necessary in order to release the psychomotor energy that has been trapped in the body. The natural flow of energy can't occur with roadblocks. A little bit of energy held somewhere in the body attracts more energy to stop at the same point. Think of the energy flow through your body as being like the blood flow through your veins. You can see how a blockage at one point can mess up the whole system's flow. Any little blockage will continue to grow and collect more stagnant energy. Beyond creating the circumstances for a healthy energy flow, this exercise addresses the flow of communication between the conscious and subconscious minds. In the first part of practice 2 in chapter 4 we touched on sending a message to the subconscious mind. Now it's time to really tune in on how that works.

It is in the stillness that powerful thoughts are developed. Stillness is a prerequisite for deep thought, powerful realizations, and growth. Have you ever noticed how you do some of your best thinking when you are still? The moments in the morning when your brain has woken up, but your body hasn't, probably produce insights or ideas that may not have come to you in another state. These happen by chance, without intention. This exercise is designed to enable you to put your body in a state of relaxation and release the held energy so that you can begin to produce these moments of clarity and insight at will. This is the first step in energy flow.

1. Begin, as before, by selecting a quiet and comfortable place to sit. It helps to be in an environment that promotes peace. It can be outside if you're lucky enough to have a space that contains nothing but the sounds of nature. If you're in a busy home, lock yourself away in a bedroom or somewhere where you won't be disturbed.

2. Sit with your back straight and self-supported—don't lean on anything. I usually sit on a bed in a cross-legged position. Rest your hands or forearms on your legs or knees. Close your eyes. With each breath in through the nose and out through the mouth, allow your muscles to relax. As you breathe in, your tummy should extend, filling your lungs from the bottom. Think of the way a puppy's tummy moves out and then relaxes with each breath when it sleeps. In the beginning you may have to tense and then relax each muscle group. This helps to build awareness of the muscles and builds that capacity to identify where you hold your tension. The "tension triangle," across the shoulders and up to the top of the head, is a common place for excess energy to be lurking. Pick up your shoulders and try to make them touch your ears as

you breathe in. Then release the breath through your mouth and allow your shoulders to drop down and back. Feel the release. Keep relaxing your body for at least fifteen minutes. This is long enough to allow you to be patient with those areas that don't want to relax. It may take time. Don't think that you're failing just because a certain area keeps its tension or brings it back immediately. This is a process.

Repeat this exercise as often as possible, preferably daily until it becomes easy to instantaneously relax every muscle in your body. At that time, you can accomplish total relaxation in any environment. In the office, at a party, or standing in line at the store, you can close your eyes for an instant, take a breath, and feel the tension leave your body.

Practice 5
EXERCISE AND BODY DISPOSITIONS

Everyone needs regular exercise. A person with psychomotor intensity has more need to keep the energy flowing outward to ensure that the channels are not stopped up. Free-flowing energy is essential to well-being and power in life.

Now that you understand the impact of different types of movement on your sense of being and your outlook on life, and you've begun to clear the energy blocks, it is clear that the type of exercise you choose can take you in many different directions. It can be used to teach your body new dispositions or reinforce some that you determine to be important.

There are five primary body dispositions: stability, flexibility, determination, openness, and centeredness. Each has its advantages in a particular time or situation. For example, the person who stays in the disposition of determination without openness being available is likely to have a hard-driving approach and experience stress when force doesn't solve a problem. A person whose body stays in flexibility will experience life feeling a little off-balance. They may get pushed and pulled with the tides. As you read these descriptions, think about which describe you and which are a little foreign to you.

STABILITY

The body position is low and stable. It feels as if there are roots connecting the body to the earth. To experience a moment of stability, try walking in place and gazing far into the distance. Keep it going for about two or three minutes. The disposition of stability contributes to the ability to stick with something. It has an eye on a distant goal, and it continues to move toward it.

FLEXIBILITY

The body position is high, even up on tiptoes. It is always moving and sometimes off-balance. It doesn't contain a feeling of control but rather a free-flowing dance. The disposition of flexibility allows creativity and improved relationships. It interacts with the world as a dance of give-and-take.

DETERMINATION

The determined body is in a forward posture. It is ready for action and adopts what looks like a fighting stance. The gaze is forward and the eyes are steady. This disposition is common in business. Determination provides for focused action. It isn't sidetracked, and it is full of power.

OPENNESS

The open body leans slightly back. It is calm and receptive. The arms are slightly lifted from the sides as if to anticipate an embrace. The disposition of openness brings the possibility for tenderness and love. It is receptive to new ideas with an absence of fear.

CENTEREDNESS

The centered body is neutral. It isn't backward, forward, up, or down. It is the place we return to from the other dispositions and allows easy movement into any disposition as needed. It is calm and alert.

Consider these five categories of disposition and the types of movement supporting each. Remember that the one you are most comfortable with, the one you are likely to choose first, is probably leaning heavily on a disposition you already have available. We all need to have each of these dispositions available. In selecting a type of exercise, I encourage you to go outside your comfort zone. Instead of reinforcing the disposition that is most comfortable to you, the one you already know and do well, this can be an opportunity to develop a new capacity. These are a few suggestions for types of exercise that can build or reinforce different dispositions.

Stability: walking, yoga, running/jogging, golf, sailing

Flexibility: dance, yoga, Pilates, surfing, skiing, gymnastics

Determination: karate, boxing, running, boot camp, weight training, football, wrestling

Openness: ballet, Qigong, Latin dance, rythmic gymnastics

Centeredness: yoga, Qigong, T'ai Chi, horseback riding

There are many other types of physical exercise. In general, you can evaluate the exercise according to the disposition it creates for you and pick the one that builds you up where you are not strong.

Important Points for the Impatient

- Practice 3: Walk a Mile in My Shoes provides a firsthand demonstration of how the way we move impacts the way we feel and think. This is a fun exercise that you will remember for years. It's also a great way to get inside someone's head and understand what it feels like to be them.

- Practice 4: Being Still and Creating Flow is an opportunity to clear out those energy blocks held in the body. In order to have the maximum ability to allow energy to flow freely, the blockages have to go. This is the first step in claiming the power of your psychomotor intense self.

- Practice 5: Exercise and Body Dispositions takes advantage of your new awareness of how movement creates different ways of thinking and feeling. Five body dispositions—stability, flexibility, determination, openness, and centeredness—are explored in terms of which kinds of movement support different possibilities in life. This is a guide to choosing a new way of moving in order to keep the energy flowing freely.

8

Intellectual Intensity

I have no special talents. I am only passionately curious.
—Albert Einstein

In the story of the ugly duckling, the differences in the way the swan looked, acted, and developed were a concern for his duckling mother and for the community of ducks. Because swans have a different developmental process and timeline than ducks, he was out of step with the group and so he was determined to be wrong in many respects. The one thing he did well, in fact better than the ducklings, was swim. It was his saving grace.

Intellectual intensity is to us like swimming was to the swan. It's the one thing we do better than the "ducks" and the one area where we receive positive feedback. It's no wonder then that we nurture this talent. The rest of our development takes its own course, which is quite different than our "duckling" friends. We now have some scientific evidence that our brains grow and mature differently than others' do. Along with that, our emotional and social skills develop differently. Now, if we were in a group of "swans," that wouldn't be an issue. We would all be within a range of normal. We are, however, raised in a society of "ducks." Now we are the ones who are out of pace with the crowd.

DIFFERENT BRAINS

Studies show that there is a distinctly different pattern of brain development in intellectually gifted people. A longitudinal study performed by the National Institutes of Mental Health (NIMH) found that children with the highest IQs developed the prefrontal cortex later than other children.[24] This latent development continued until about eleven years of age, at which point they had thicker, denser cortical matter than their less intelligent same-age peers. They then very quickly completed the pruning process to end up with brains that appear to be similar to the brains of normal children in size and thickness or density.[25]

We also know that early stimulation, identical to sensual intensity, causes development of cognitive functioning in addition to emotional, behavioral, motor, and social development. If sensual stimulation is causative for brain development, it stands to reason that it could be playing a part in intellectual intensity.[26] In an experiment conducted at the University of Illinois, rats raised in a sensually rich environment developed up to 25 percent more synapses per nerve cell.[27]

Intellectual intensity is created by a brain that works differently. Picture the brain of a nonintense person as a highway system with roads leading to other roads. Thoughts travel these well-maintained and structured pathways. New roads are designed and built, providing access to new information as it is categorized and stored. The more often the roads are traveled, the wider they become and the more accessible the information stored along that road. Now picture the intense brain as something more like the Internet, with new connections made very quickly, resulting in a network that can appear messy and confusing. These two different approaches to thinking are sometimes called linear and nonlinear thinking. Linear thinking is described as being rational, logical, and analytical. Nonlinear thinking is more intuitive, creative, and insightful. Intense people lean toward the nonlinear style of thinking. That doesn't mean that we aren't logical or analytical. It does mean that we are able to use intuition within analysis.

INTELLECTUAL INTENSITY AND INTELLIGENCE

While intellectually intense people are most certainly gifted, it may not be reflected in an IQ test. Intellectual intensity is more a quality of how a person learns and thinks than it is about IQ. IQ tests really measure two things, "fluid intelligence" and "crystallized intelligence." Fluid intelligence is the ability to solve problems in novel situations. It doesn't rely as much on knowledge that has already been acquired, but instead uses the ability to think in the here and now. It still requires logic and analysis but doesn't depend on information already stored about the situation. Crystallized intelligence is the ability to use what has already been learned and stored. It is more likely to change as we gain education and experience throughout life. Intellectually intense people will likely score high in fluid intelligence due to the way an intense brain works through association and patterns. The crystallized intelligence score may vary depending on the person's cultural, social, and educational exposures. Basically, for the person whose fluid intelligence is stronger than their crystallized intelligence, it's easier to figure out something new than it is to memorize and retrieve information. This preference for figuring things out leads to a different method of thinking.

LEARNING AND THINKING PATTERNS

We take information in differently. For the nonlinear thinker, the act of thinking about something causes it to be stored in memory. Because we think about what interests us, we more easily learn about things that are closely associated with something else we find interesting, something that causes an emotional response, or something that is unusual or novel. Because much of our learning is driven by interest, the process is sometimes a feverish pursuit of information. At some point in the process, the subject is completely absorbed. We call this embodying the information. It becomes a part of us. We also take in information outside of our areas of interest because of the lenient gatekeeper. The gatekeeper allows more information and experience to pass through to consciousness. In some cases children are fully aware of the subject matter being taught in school before any formal education has been supplied. A casual exposure to new ideas and concepts results in information coming in and being stored. The result is a network that stores more information with looser structure.

This Internet type of brain uses a function much like a web browser to retrieve information. A question can be proposed, causing a wide search of the information that has been fully embodied. Similarities are sought out in one of many facets. One of the many advantages of this structure is that it allows connections to be made between seemingly unrelated subjects. For example the search may return a result where the pattern is similar, but the subject is completely different. Like the results returned from a web browser, there are many results from which to choose.

Schools are designed to teach the nonintense type of brain, the linear thinking style. They use practice and repetition to create the pathways in order to store the information. The nonintense child is well adapted to this approach for learning. The intense child is only frustrated by it. When a math teacher insists on seeing the "work" behind the answer to a question, he is looking for evidence that the child has built and traveled the correct roads in order to store the information. For the intense child, the road is not nearly as concrete.

They may intuitively know answers and not be able to "show" their work because there wasn't any.

KEY TRAITS OF INTELLECTUAL INTENSITY

This intellectual pattern has a few key traits, most of which are familiar to the intellectually intense person. We learn quickly in areas of interest. We are eternally curious, sometimes perfectionists, and do not tolerate boredom very well at all. While we love ideas and problem solving, we can appear scattered when following one interest to the next and to the next.

Quick Learner

The intellectually intense person is quick to grasp ideas and eager to learn in their areas of interest. They are able to understand concepts at a deeper level than most. Although they may recognize that they learn more quickly than others, they often don't consider themselves gifted.

In *Enjoying the Gift of Being Uncommon*, Willem Kuipers describes the signs of what he refers to as "XIP," or extra intelligent person, with five characteristics:

1. Intellectually able

2. Incurably inquisitive

3. Needs autonomy

4. Excessive zeal in pursuit of interests

5. Contrast between intellectual and emotional self-confidence[28]

He claims that a person who recognizes three of the five characteristics in themselves is XIP. Note that this description doesn't depend on an IQ score, or even strictly on intelligence. He alternates the meaning of XIP between "extra intelligent person" and "extra intense person." He also explains in some detail how the XIP person rarely considers him or herself as extra intelligent and is more comfortable with the alternate meaning of extra intensity.

Kuipers brings up an interesting aspect of intellectual intensity, which is the tendency for these people to reject or at least doubt a label of "gifted" or "highly intelligent." He cites several possible reasons for this, but the reason that makes the most sense to me is the one that coincides with Dabrowski's view of the intense person being filled with feelings of inferiority and self-doubt. If the intense person can identify someone else who has a greater mastery over a subject, then by comparison, her own knowledge is insufficient. If she has a sibling who is identified as gifted, then by comparison, she is not. If she performs sporadically in school, succeeding in some areas and failing in others, then she feels that she can't possibly be gifted. And most prominently, the failure to perform according to her own ideals provides constant proof of her shortcomings.

Curiosity

Curiosity is another common thread in intellectual intensity. What we may consider to be childlike curiosity remains in adults with intellectual intensity. Things that others take for granted such as how things work or societal values can be sparks for intense study and analysis. The study of complex systems or concepts is a source of excitement. Insatiable curiosity combined with an ability to learn and understand quickly and deeply creates a mind where relationships between things are multifaceted. Simple answers are rejected in favor of more intricate explanations that take into account the complex nature of the world. These complex people are more able to hold multiple sides of the same argument as possibilities.

Perfectionism

Perfectionism is common with intellectual intensity. The ideal in one's mind of what should be never matches up with what is, and it creates a lot of doubt and self-flagellation. Helpful hints are available everywhere. Such words of wisdom as "learn to accept that good enough is acceptable" or "set realistic goals" are the result of looking at perfectionism from the outside, as though it is an attribute of someone else. However, when perfectionism is lived personally, these bits of advice sound hollow.

A better approach is to learn to apply perfectionism in the areas where it provides the most important possibilities, and to let it go in those areas that really don't matter. This is covered in more detail in chapter 15.

Love of Ideas, Theories, Analysis, and Problem Solving

Intellectual intensity reveals itself in a love of thinking and everything associated with it. New ideas and theories are as welcome and necessary as air, food, or water. To have a big intellectual problem to solve is to be happy. The flexibility of thought patterns allowed by the looser structure in the intense brain means that it is possible to scan for information to enable problem solving in much the same way we might browse the Internet. Anything that has some similarity is returned even if it isn't in the same subject area. Patterns are recognized across disciplines and used creatively. Using our brains the way they seem to have been intended is joyful.

Being Scattered in Too Many Directions

Natural curiosity combined with a quick mind results in varied interests. It's normal for an intellectually intense person to be watching television, researching something on the Internet, and having a telephone conversation at the same time. Many have two or three books going at once. Add to that the natural tendency for the intense mind to have loose associations, and you have a recipe for scattered thought and conversation patterns.

Open an email, and there's a link to some interesting article. While reading that you notice an ad on the right with some outrageous claim, so outrageous that you just have to click through to see what it's about. Then you find a term you don't understand, so you look that up. And on it goes. A quick check of email can take a person on a "three-hour cruise" driven by interest after interest after interest. Like the lost souls on Gilligan's Island, they may never return to the original port of call.

Low Tolerance for Boredom

The intense brain has to be busy. Boredom is the ultimate enemy. This is impossible to explain to a nonintense person. Boredom is torture. When bored, even some pretty stupid things start to look like good ideas. My firstborn son decided, at six years old, that he would cure his boredom at school one day by crawling under the desks of the other children and tying their shoelaces together. I'm convinced that at least half of what we call impulsivity is really a desperate attempt to break free from boredom.

Without an interesting pastime, we turn to entertainment or information gathering. Television is an easy way to temporarily escape boredom. For a little while we are soothed by the TV taking over with a slow pace and mindless content. Video games are more interactive but still lack any form of real intellectual stimulation.

Constant information gathering through surfing the net or reading books or newspapers is another boredom fighter.

Basically anything is preferable to boredom, and our boredom relievers may or may not serve us. Not that we have to be productive all the time, but the habitual methods we find to relieve boredom can take over and prevent us from tackling anything deeper. While entertainment and information gathering may keep us from our enemy of boredom, they don't always provide the nourishment our minds really need. As Tryon Edwards said, "Contemplation is to knowledge what digestion is to food—the way to get life out of it."

CHALLENGES OF INTELLECTUAL INTENSITY

Intellectual intensity is not without its challenges. Having brains that work differently impacts almost every area of life, but nothing is more strongly affected than our relationships. Our thought patterns, being more complex and diverse than those of our nonintense friends and family, can lead to frustrations for all concerned.

Moving Too Quickly

In conversation, one of the most common characteristics of intellectual intensity is moving from one subject to the next as we follow the intricate associations in our brains. These perceived changes of subject are confusing and sometimes frustrating to a less intense person trying to keep up. The connection between one subject and the next, while obvious to us, sometimes leaves the other person behind, bewildered by our ramblings.

Sometimes information comes to us so quickly that others can't understand how we do it. The capacity to take in and retrieve information quickly can intimidate others. It can cause them to be a little uncomfortable because they don't understand it. It can even cause them to be suspicious or distrustful. We are different in so many ways that people often don't understand us, and as a result they quite naturally feel unable to predict our actions. An inability to predict is threatening. When a person senses that you may be much smarter than they, the need to understand your moral character becomes very important. A smart person who is kind and caring is much less threatening than a smart person who doesn't really care about other people. Any slight indication of less-than-perfect morals is amplified due to your perceived intellectual power. This can cause people to take seemingly unwarranted shots at us. There is a desire to knock us down a bit. This is particularly true when the less intense person is in a position of authority over you or has an assessment that they "should" be smarter or better than you. To an intense person, these undeserved attacks only serve to distance us further. Introverts become more introverted. Extroverts become bolder.

The Trap of "Figuring It Out"

Another potential pitfall of intellectual intensity is derived from the confidence we have in our ability to think. Thinking works, problem solving is fruitful and enjoyable, and figuring it out is a natural strength that we recognize and use heavily. We have found such success with intellectual pursuits that we lean too heavily on "figuring it out," regardless of the nature of the problem. The tendency to intellectualize emotional subjects or problems has two primary outcomes. First, since "figuring it out" doesn't work in the emotional domain, the exercise is a waste of time and energy. The failure can cause further emotional distress and feelings of helplessness. Second, the intellectual approach to emotional issues serves to support others' assessment of our character as cold and heartless. "Figuring it out" also doesn't work with aesthetic pursuits, although that doesn't stop a lot of people from trying it.

Stupid People

The single biggest challenge I hear about from intellectually intense people is the self-induced emotional distress brought on by "stupid" people. There seems to be nothing else that hits the same triggers. Emotional reactions including anger and frustration are common. The same self-doubt and perfectionism that cause us to reject a label of "gifted" or "genius" also cause us to believe that everyone ought to be able to think and learn the way we do. When an intense person can more quickly understand something, or when you can naturally predict a likely outcome from a suggested action, it comes so easily that it seems that others should be able to do the same. It's very difficult to understand that what comes easily to you may be extremely difficult for others. With very few exceptions, we tend to lump everyone into the "same as me" category. Using that logic, if they are the same as you, and you can figure it out, then they must have some other motive. We attribute some questionable or downright evil motive to the actions of the so-called stupid person that is the true trigger for our own anger or frustration. Do you remember a time when you were upset, even to the point of true anger, over the stupid actions of another person? Do you become enraged by "stupid" drivers? Are you prone to this kind of suffering on a regular basis?

Relationships: We Really Are Different

The relationship challenges associated with intellectual intensity are all based in a lack of understanding of the differences between intense and nonintense ways of thinking, learning and behaving. First is a need to thoroughly understand ourselves. Recognizing how the way our intense brains work allows us to recognize when we are intellectualizing and when we are traveling too fast in conversation. Understanding how we are different than others sheds light on the effect we may have on them, how we may be perceived as threatening, and how we may be prone to generalizing any behavior that frustrates us as stupid. Understanding is the first step toward relieving the suffering and separateness we feel with others. With each intensity, the path to relieving the suffering and developing the intensity is first to understand it. The second step is to do the practices. The third step is to have support along the way.

Gear Shifter

Finally, a common challenge for the intellectually intense is difficulty shifting attention from one subject or one activity to another. This is known as the gear shifter of the brain. In intense brains the gear shifter isn't under as much conscious control as it is in less intense brains. You'd think shifting would be easy given the way we can jump from subject to subject, but the reality is that those jumps are driven by interest. Without interest to drive a shift, we tend to dally too long on one thing. For example, if I have a list of tasks to get done, I will work on the first one, sometimes to completion, but moving on to the second task is quite difficult. It takes an enormous amount of energy to simply move from task to task. This is almost impossible to explain to nonintense people.

INTENSITY AND VALUE SYSTEMS

The way the intense brain works to take in information, store it, and retrieve it is only a part of the story. What we do with that information and how we use it to make decisions and judgments about the world around us are determined by the internal map of reality. The biggest influence on the internal map is our value system. The values we hold dear act as a magnet for beliefs, thoughts, and ideas. They form the structure by which we view and act within the world.

You may have noticed that as you grew up, your values changed. Through a natural process, we incorporate new values while rejecting a few of the older ones. For most people the growth process continues until they reach a set of values that matches their family and the culture in which they live. For others the growth process continues. Intensity sets us up for a continued growth process. In part because of the way our brains work to soak up information, supported by creativity and the anxiety that keeps us from becoming too settled in our ways, we are more likely to grow beyond our immediate environments.

This growth of values is not as arbitrary as you might imagine. We tend to think of values as a list. It seems as if there are an almost limitless number of values out there and people have a random selection that makes up their personal value system. It's as though there were an a la carte menu of values we select from to form our own very personalized combination. In truth, the selection is more like picking a complete meal of values from a very short list of options. To add to the predictability, each meal is taken in a predetermined order. We all start with the first selection and progress through them in order until we're full and we stop. The only significant variation is the stopping point.

Dr. Clare Graves, professor of psychology at Union College, spent his life studying value systems and discovered this surprising truth about the predictable growth in values and the way values influence thoughts, ideas, and beliefs. He found that there were two parts to the influence. One is the way we see the world; the other is how we cope within that view of the world. This work has been taken up by Don Beck and Chris Cowan, who further developed Dr. Graves's theory into what is now known as Spiral Dynamics.[29]

The name refers to the way Dr. Graves envisioned this pattern of development as a spiral. He actually saw it as a double helix, like DNA. One strand was the view of the world at a certain level, and the corresponding strand was the method of coping attached to that particular view of the world. It was viewed as a spiral because as one progresses through the value systems, there is a tendency to revisit previous places but at a new level. In order to make the system easier to understand, Beck and Cowan dumped the double helix explanation and replaced it with random colors representing each level.

VALUE LEVELS OF DEVELOPMENT

Color	Map of Reality	Methods to Cope	Intensity
Beige	The world is a state of nature and biological urges and drives: physical senses dictate the state of being	Use instincts	Sensual intensity reigns in infancy
Purple	The world is threatening and full of mysterious powers and spirit beings that must be placated and appeased	Use tradition and ritual— a tribal approach	Imagination blossoms in toddlerhood— fantasy
Red	The world is like a jungle where the tough and strong prevail, and the weak serve; nature is an adversary to be conquered	Use power, attempt to dominate or align self with the more powerful for protection	Emotional intensity—strong sense of self— terrible twos

Color	Map of Reality	Methods to Cope	Intensity
Blue	The world is controlled by a higher power that punishes evil and eventually rewards good works and righteous living	Do what is "right," follow the rules, conform, don't stand out	Intensity is disorder
Orange	The world is full of resources to develop and opportunities to make things better and bring prosperity	Achieve results and get ahead, innovate, shine, or some will cheat	Intensity is an asset, emotional sensitivity may cause suffering
Green	The world is the habitat wherein humanity can find life and purposes through affiliation and sharing	Respond to human needs, work cooperatively, stand up for causes	Emotional sensitivity is an asset
Yellow	The world is a chaotic organism where change is the norm and uncertainty an acceptable state of being	Live and let live, learn systemic interdependence, appreciate value of all previous levels	Intellectual intensity is the biggest asset, other intensities are valued
Turquoise	The world is a delicately balanced system of interlocking forces in jeopardy at humanity's hands; chaordic	Collective consciousness, interconnected, transpersonal, collaborate	Intensity finds company with other intense beings

(continues)

(continued)

Color	Map of Reality	Methods to Cope	Intensity
Coral	Too soon to say but the world should be I-oriented, controlling, consolidating	Too soon to say	Too soon to say
Teal	The world is a return to we-oriented	Too soon to say	Too soon to say

Not only individuals but also groups of people go through these value levels. Organizations, societies, even countries go through these levels as they progress. There is an interesting dynamic between the value level of the individual and the value level of the organizations they belong to and the larger society in which they live. If you've ever worked in an organization that seemed wrong to you on many levels, that was most likely a mismatch between your value level and that of the organization.

Beige

We all start at the beige level. Beige is about survival. The world is a dangerous place. The individual uses instincts to survive. All babies come into the world at this level. They cry when they need attention and have little to no awareness of self as separate from the world. An adult at a beige level would be primarily concerned with biological urges such as sex and hunger.

At each level there is a breakdown that can create the motivation to move to the next level. This breakdown is actually recognition that the internal map of reality doesn't adequately match reality. Moving from one level to the next is a falling apart of the internal map of reality and rebuilding it again at a higher level. At beige the breakdown is one of having no explanation for the world. When a baby realizes that there is a separation between self and the world, there is a need to understand that difference.

Purple

Purple is a view of the world as a sort of magical place. With no understanding of natural laws or an explanation for why things happen as they do, a view forms of a mystical place where some beings have power and others do not. One must placate the powerful by use of rituals. In children, this is the time when they recognize that their parents are all-powerful. One of my sons asked if Grandma made the sun and the moon go up and down. I suppose she was seen as the all-mighty goddess.

The eventual breakdown in purple is a desire to have one's own power. As we go through the breakdowns, we may reject a part of the value system, but for the most part it's retained. We just add on to it with the next level. If you doubt that you have retained any of the purple value system, ask yourself if you have a lucky shirt you wear whenever your sports team is playing. Do you have any rituals that you perform for fear of something bad happening if you don't, just in case? Even though you understand rationally that a certain ritual or lucky charm can't make a difference, that part of you that still believes is alive and well.

Red

Red is all about power. Of course the aim here is to have power. There is a shunning of sources of power recognized in purple. No more goddesses, no more parental rule. This is the birth of the terrible twos. It's an "all about me" level where one takes as much as possible. The view of the world is shifted to a place where power gets the spoils. Since a fine-tuned sense of right and wrong comes in a later value system, anything goes. As such, power can be won or lost in a flash.

As I mentioned before, these value levels are mirrored in societies and countries around the world. Although we aren't normally aware of societies in beige and purple, we do see red playing a part in world politics. A country in the red value system will have a dictator, or more likely a series of dictators, with ultimate power and little regard for the people they rule over. Because of the volatility of this set of values, the balance of power shifts as soon as another is positioned to take over. There are coups and a definite lack of structure and predictability, which is the breakdown in red. Whether in an organization, a country, or a person, the lack of stability and the distrust that prevail at this level become intolerable.

Blue

Blue is the answer to the chaos in red. In blue the world is a place of hierarchy. Everyone has a place, a function, and a role to perform. Most importantly, there is order. This level makes a distinction between good and evil as a primary determinant in action. The call is to decide what is right and good and then force that. The world is seen as being ruled by a higher power that rewards good deeds and punishes evil. The method of coping in this world is to conform and follow the rules. There is a sense of honor when performing good deeds. As a society, a blue value system may still have a dictator, but they enforce order instead of chaos. We see examples of a blue culture in the military, law enforcement, healthcare, most educational systems, and organizations such as scouting and organized religion. Virtually any organization in uniform values and enforces conformity.

The breakdown in blue comes when the need for self-expression, innovation, or freedom of thought overpowers the need to conform. In addition to those issues, there is a special kind of breakdown in the blue value system for the intense person. Because blue values include doing what is expected, predictability in actions, following the rules, and prohibiting thinking for yourself to some extent, intense people are at a distinct disadvantage. We are by nature different. And different is bad in blue. It is for this reason that intensity is labeled as a disorder. When the only options to categorize differences are viewing them as either evil or sick, disorder seems the lesser label to wear. This is a difficult time. The true strengths of intensity are devalued at this level, and the weaknesses are exaggerated. We assess ourselves as broken in some way and feel helpless. I've heard coaching clients in blue suffer terribly over the inability to behave predictably over time.

Orange

Orange is a return to the focus on self we saw in the red level. This time, the self has been tamed by the virtues learned in the blue value system. Once released from the overwhelming structure in blue, the individual is free to direct their own path. The world is seen as being full of resources to be used in order to create prosperity. At this level individual accomplishments are expected to bring individual rewards. Possessions are seen as proof of self-worth. We cope within orange by striving to get ahead.

Innovation, creativity, intelligence, and cunning are all valued. Luckily for the intense person, we have all those things in abundance. This is the level at which intensity turns to a real asset. Those who have embraced their intensity may refer to ADHD as the CEO disorder. They wear it as a badge. It is proof of the differences that make them great. The person who is at an orange level and working within an orange organization is likely to be successful. The intense person who is at orange and working within orange is likely to be wildly successful.

But at some point all the striving and success become hollow. The crisis at this transition is one of meaning. There grows a longing for purpose beyond the shallow accumulation of things and increasing symbols of success.

Green

Green is the level of causes, purpose, and passion. When searching for a purpose, we will most definitely find one. Whether it is to save the planet or feed the hungry, something will appear that lights a fire in the soul. The hunger for meaning in orange is fulfilled by deeply felt causes in green. The sensitivity that comes with intensity, particularly emotional sensitivity, fuels this value level. We are passionate and sensitive to the struggles of others. We care deeply, and in this way, intense people find some sense of validation in green. This level marks a return to the focus on ourselves as a part of a whole as it was in blue, but this time we're calling the shots. The class system in blue is seen as too predetermined and the ruthlessness of the struggle in orange as too cutthroat. A system that ensures equality and fair treatment for all is the only answer. Greenpeace and other environmental groups, Whole Foods Market, John Lennon's music, and Doctors without Borders are all examples of green organizations and messages.

The concept of equality in green extends far beyond sharing of resources. It embraces the concept that all views should be honored. It goes to great lengths to avoid holding one person above another, one faith above another, or one opinion above all others, in theory anyway. This creates a problem when it becomes difficult to take any sort of stand without devaluing some other opinion. If we are all equal, and our stands all have some sort of value, how can one be better than another? This level begins to feel burdensome. There is an overwhelming sense of responsibility combined with the powerlessness that comes from the inability to step on any toes. While we aren't likely to abandon the purpose we found in green, it's entirely possible to become so fed up with the approach that we go in search of something better.

Yellow

The move to the yellow value level marks a milestone in this view of value development. Beige through green are considered to be the first tier. Yellow, being the first step within the second tier, corresponds to beige. It is self-focused, as was beige, but this time the infant is figurative. We are like an infant in a new view of an entirely new world. We see the connections between living things and desire to understand the complexity. We study for the sake of learning itself and are fascinated with complexity, living systems, and the interconnectedness of all things. This broader view of the world has a very nice side effect. Because we no longer identify ourselves with our possessions, because we are beginning to see the connectedness of all life, very little appears as a threat. We are rarely afraid. The emphasis in yellow on knowledge and competency creates the perfect Petri dish for the full expression of intellectual intensity. We rarely find organizations operating at a yellow level, since this is so rare. Only about 1 percent of the world population is thought to be at a yellow value level.

The breakdown at yellow can be assumed to be a greater desire to be within the world and more connected. Given the focus on education, a move to turquoise would be a logical next step to begin sharing the knowledge gained.

Although three more levels have been named, there is too little information about them to define the world view, the coping methods, or the breakdowns that would cause a move to the next level.

Important Points for the Impatient

- Intellectual intensity is about the way a person thinks and learns, not about IQ. It is a nonlinear type of functioning that includes a desire to keep the mind moving, perfectionism, curiosity, and following your interests.

- If we don't develop intellectual intensity, we're likely to feed it with junk food of the mind. Junk food consists of collecting facts, playing games, watching TV, or any other activity that keeps the mind busy without challenging it.

- Intellectual intensity is one of three key components required to continue to develop an advanced system of values. The development of value systems is a predictable developmental process.

- In only one of these value levels, intensity is often considered a disorder. Escape from that value system means the end of viewing yourself as disordered and the beginning of a journey wherein intensity is an asset.

9

Intellectual Practices: Building Intellectual Muscle

The great end of education is to discipline rather than to furnish the mind; to train it to the use of its own powers, rather than fill it with the accumulation of others.

—TRYON EDWARDS

The purpose of developing intellectual intensity is, as Tryon Edwards indicates, to discipline the considerable powers of mind found in the intellectually intense. These practices are intended to be done repeatedly over time until you see a remarkable improvement in your ability to pay attention, concentrate, and contemplate. These are skills, just like learning to play the piano, and there's no magic pill to produce the results. Practice is the only method by which the skills are learned and perfected.

Attention, concentration, and contemplation are available to everyone but are particularly useful for intellectually intense people because of the complexity of our minds. They are imperative if you want to fully use the gift of intellectual intensity. I argued in chapter 2 that the most successful managers and companies concentrated their energy on developing the strengths of their best employees. The same concept applies here. While intellectual intensity is already considered a strength for most, further development of this area yields the most powerful results. There are four intellectual practices in this chapter. Practice 6, The Magic Word, develops the power of attention. Practice 7, Concentration on a Subject, develops concentration. Practice 8, The Lost Art, develops contemplation. We can be masters of our own minds. Finally, if you find that your value level is causing problems, particularly if you are having problems seeing your intensity as the gift that it is, practice 9, Value Development and Growth, is about moving to the next value level.

Practice 6
THE MAGIC WORD

The range of attention for intense people is off the scale at both ends of the spectrum. We can be incredibly inattentive or hyperfocused. Instead of the level of attention happening at random, this exercise will enable you choose. You will be able to bring your mind to attention at will. It can only be at a pure attentional state when it is in the present moment in its current surroundings. If the mind is busy in the past, the future, or some other imagined place, it isn't here, now. I have no reason to deny the mind its fantasies. Creative intensity is all about that. This is an exercise to develop the ability of the mind to attend to what is in front of it in the present moment in time and the existing situation. The surprise with this exercise is that the present isn't nearly as boring as you would think if you're really completely in it. It's when you're half in and half out that it seems dull. Reality, right here and right now, is actually full of fascinating experiences.

1. Find a magic word for yourself. Any word will do. Just for fun I'll use "kablam." There are those who recommend something much more literal like "Be here now." That's fine too.

2. Now imagine that thinking the word "kablam" endows the thinker with magical powers of attention. Whenever I think the word, I am reminded that I am going to be completely present to the object of my attention. If I am talking with someone and my mind begins to drift, a simple "kablam" repeated in my mind returns my attention to the person in front of me. I am back. I am completely present and engaged with that person. I really watch their facial expressions and attend to the conversation. The goal here is just to be in the present moment. Thoughts of the past or worries about the future can be postponed. If you are particularly hesitant to give up those thoughts, allow yourself a specific time each day to indulge to your heart's desire in the past and the future. But don't allow those thoughts to take over when you're being present.

This practice will be challenging at first. Don't let that discourage you. You will get better at it. If you give yourself a goal to practice being present for two weeks, you'll make noticeable progress. Remember that the goal of the exercise is to gain mastery over how you use your mind. In learning any new skill, we go through the stages of unconscious incompetence, conscious incompetence, conscious competence, and finally unconscious competence.

Unconscious incompetence is the stage you may have been at before the realization that you were not using your mind to its fullest.

Conscious incompetence is the stage where you have an idea of a level of attention that is possible along with the awareness that you are not able to achieve it, or if achieved, you realize that you are not able to maintain it for long. You begin to notice patterns of thoughts that distract you. Certain themes of mulling over the past, worry about the future, or dreams of things to come will repeat themselves. Your mind has its own version of multitasking, called multithinking. It has a frantic pace sometimes, never lighting on one thought for long, as the next thought carries with it a sense of urgency to be entertained.

Conscious competence will come after practice. You'll begin to see that you can be present when you choose. Your magic word will help here. It serves to bring you back to the present when you drift. During this stage you'll need the magic word less often. You'll also notice that you are better able to appreciate and enjoy life. Those moments when you are completely "in the flow," when you are completely involved in what you are doing, when you don't even notice the passage of time, become more common. Food tastes better. Friends are more enjoyable. Even mundane tasks like housework are fun when you aren't also worrying or somehow living through the past or future in your mind.

Unconscious competence may arrive one day. I can't speak with any authority of this stage of being present. I believe that I've been present for most of one day, one time. I'm told that some Zen monks have achieved this on an ongoing basis. In *One Taste*, Ken Wilber describes his experiences of being completely in this state for days and nights at a time.

Practice 7

CONCENTRATION ON A SUBJECT

Concentration is not generally taught in school. It's expected that students come pre-equipped with the ability to concentrate. There's a difference between being able to stay on task, even in a boring subject, and the skill of concentration. Less intense and less intellectual people have a much easier time staying on task than we do. It looks on the outside as if they have superior abilities for concentration. I would argue that they just don't get bored as easily. But real concentration, the ability to take an idea, consider it from all sides, compare it to currently held concepts and beliefs, and find its merits and pitfalls is rare. Far from being boring, it can be fascinating.

You've undoubtedly experienced intense concentration. There are times when the rest of the world seems to vanish and the only thing remaining is the subject of your attention. You're already familiar with the feeling, the rush, and the unbridled joy of intense concentration. Building it as a skill involves having more control over when you concentrate and on which subject, person, concept, and so on.

This type of concentration is an exercise in focus on a single subject. It is, very simply, sitting with eyes closed and concentrating on a single subject. It can include a review and questioning of what is known on the subject, consideration of other views, identifying aspects of the subject that are not known, an objective review of your emotional reaction to the subject, and other perspectives.

1. Select a subject worthy of concentration. It can be a problem that is currently vexing you, a project you would like to do, a relationship, or anything else of significant complexity. Concentrating on simple things is more advanced. Let's start with a subject with enough complexity to keep your mind busy for several minutes.

2. Simply sit still in a relaxed position but with a straight back. Close your eyes. Allow your body to relax as in practice 4, Being Still and Creating Flow, in chapter 5. When your body is relaxed, begin to think about your subject. Your mind will wander. When it does, gently return to your subject of concentration. Admonishing yourself for having wandered is just another distraction. There is no need to try to push the distraction away. To do so will only reinforce it. It works like this: Don't think of an elephant. Whatever you do, don't think about an elephant lumbering up to you and reaching out with

its trunk to touch your hand. You can't help but think of that elephant, right? It's the same way when trying to get rid of a distraction. Your focus on the distraction by trying to push it out of your mind only serves to anchor it there. Instead, just calmly return to the subject of your concentration. Welcome it back. Do this for about ten minutes. Then it's time to move on to practice 8, which fosters contemplation.

Practice 8
THE LOST ART OF CONTEMPLATION

Contemplation is not normally even on the radar in any formal educational system. Contemplation is defined as a long and thoughtful consideration. There are many contemplation practices, some of which are associated with religious traditions. The kind of contemplation I'm referring to is not a religious practice. It's a method of thinking that produces a different quality of thought. This is deep, reflective thought, which brings a profound understanding of a subject and often produces insight and new levels of awareness.

For this exercise, we continue from the end of practice 8. Since the mind is primed with a subject, it is ready to go into a freewheeling kind of state that allows deeper insights about the subject to surface.

1. After ten minutes or so of concentration, while still seated with your eyes closed, allow your mind to go blank. Check back in to be sure your body is still in a relaxed state.

2. Now just breathe. Using your breath as a focal point, breathe in and breathe out. Keep your focus on your breathing. Thoughts will continue to come to your attention. If they are not on the subject of your contemplation, let them pass by. Go back to your breath. Only allow those thoughts related to

your subject to linger. When a related thought is played out, go back to your breath again awaiting the next one.

3. This is quiet and calm time when nothing is demanded of you. There is nothing to do, there is nothing to think. Just be. This is when the subconscious mind has an opportunity to speak. Deep insights are available just below the surface of the conscious mind. They come in pictures, thoughts, or emotions. Whatever happens is just fine. There is no need to judge this communication. There is no worry about if you're "doing it right." Just breathe and be. Whatever happens is perfect.

Practice 9
VALUE DEVELOPMENT AND GROWTH

If earlier in the chapter you determined your value level, and see in that the source of your suffering, you can move on to the next level. Intellectual, creative, and emotional intensities form a dynamic trio involved in moving from one value level to another. The part played by intellectual intensity is becoming curious about the next value level; the emotional and creative elements are covered later. We naturally progress though the spiral by being immersed in the next level. The very same dynamic can cause us to stagnate at the level we reach in adulthood. The influences of family, peer group, and profession are strong enough to create either a pull to the next level or a force to stay at the current level. I'm not advocating dumping your family, friends, or job. Being aware of the influence they exert on your developmental level is enough. What is needed is an expansion.

In order to expand your awareness to the next level, immersion is the best route. While immersion doesn't really lend itself to a predetermined set of steps, as other practices have used, it can still be accomplished. Immersion is the natural path of progression to the next value level and it is aided by intensity. In order to immerse yourself in the next value level, you must find it within society.

Some levels are better represented within society due to the simple fact that more people are within that level. As higher levels are reached, finding entire communities within those levels is difficult, but not impossible. To immerse yourself in a level that isn't readily available to you within your family or community, try reading books. While immersion provides the vision of the next level, quiet contemplative practices, such as the ones presented here or more traditional meditation, provide the ability to release the current level.

The summaries below of where to find communities of each value level, and the values to be mastered, begin with blue. Beige, purple, and red are not included since adults would be expected to be at least at a red level. Only children go through the early stages, and their families provide enough immersion in higher levels to allow their development to happen naturally up to at least the red level. Most of the civilized world rests between blue and orange.

BLUE

The blue level represents 40 percent of the world population and 30 percent of the power. It is found in the military, most educational institutions, authoritarian democracies, some corporations, religion, scouting, and any order wearing uniforms. Values to be mastered in blue include honor, loyalty, principles of right and wrong, awareness of a higher power, and the effect behavior has on the group.

ORANGE

The orange level represents 30 percent of the world population and 50 percent of the power. It is found in most of the corporate world, Wall Street, and multiparty democracies. Values to be mastered in orange include welcoming change and innovation, scientific analysis, competition as a means for improvement, individualism, experimentation, rational logic, and strategy.

GREEN

The green level represents 10 percent of the world population and 15 percent of the power. It is found in ecology movements, humanistic psychology, social democracies, Greenpeace, animal rights, human rights, cultural creatives, and the New Age movement. Values to be mastered in green include equality and fairness, consensus, harmony, spirituality, diversity, multiculturalism, and caring for the Earth.

YELLOW

The yellow level represents 1 percent of the world population and 5 percent of the power. It is found in integral psychology, Ken Wilber's *A Theory of Everything* and *One Taste*, Integral Transformative Practice International (*www.itp-life.com*), and Robert Kegan's *In over Our Heads*.

Values and concepts to be mastered in yellow include flexibility, autonomy, natural hierarchy, self-worth, existentialism, systems, interdependence, questioning, and integration.

TURQUOISE

The turquoise level represents less that 0.1 percent of the world population and 1 percent of the power. It is not found in many places. I would look to the centers mentioned in yellow, since yellow is the beginning of the second tier of being. Values and concepts to master in turquoise include interconnectedness, collective consciousness, survival of life on Earth, transpersonal concept of reality, and holism.

A NOTE ON THE PRACTICES SO FAR

There have been a lot of practices suggested thus far, and it may seem overwhelming at this point. Since so many of the practices include some sort of meditation or contemplation, I recommend that you become familiar with the practices and choose the one that works best for you. Doing any sort of quiet reflective practice will help to develop all the intensities. The practices in this chapter differ from the others, as they are designed specifically to develop your ability to think deeply with focus. There are many more practices to come. One is sure to strike your fancy.

Important Points for the Impatient

- Attention is nothing more than being completely present in this place at this time. We learn in Practice 6 that a word or phrase can be used to return wandering attention to the present.

- Concentration is a powerful mental tool that is easier to master than one might think. Practice 7: Concentration on a Subject teaches the discipline of concentrating at will.

- Building on concentration, Practice 8: The Lost Art of Contemplation, begins the conversation between the conscious and subconscious minds.

- Practice 9: Value Development and Growth provides the foundation needed to move to the next value level. For those who have determined that a part of their suffering is related to the value level in which they dwell.

10

Creative Intensity

*The truly creative mind in any field is no more than this: A
human creature born abnormally, inhumanly sensitive. To
him . . . a touch is a blow, a sound is a noise, a misfortune
is a tragedy, a joy is an ecstasy, a friend is a lover, a lover is a
god, and failure is death. Add to this cruelly delicate organ-
ism the overpowering necessity to create, create, create—so that
without the creating of music or poetry or books or buildings
or something of meaning, his very breath is cut off from him.
He must create, must pour out creation. By some strange,
unknown, inward urgency he is not really alive unless he is
creating.*

—PEARL S. BUCK

Creativity is the most elusive of the intensities. Ask an intense person if they are creative and you are likely to strike a chord. Some
will have already decided that they deserve the title. They may feign
humility while admitting that others have labeled them as creative.
Others will boldly accept all that the word implies. Still others will
shy away from it—either because they truly believe that they are
not at all creative or because they think that whatever it is that they
do isn't worthy of the title "creative." I suppose this charmed quality of the concept of creativity stems from a medieval belief that all

creativity was in the domain of God. "Creativity" meant to create from nothing and it was generally accepted that only God could create from nothing. The mere mortal could only imitate. Since then definitions and concepts of creativity have become more inclusive. Poetry, visual arts, storytelling and performance arts, among others are now viewed as having the inspiration and imagination required to classify as creativity. Whether a creative act is proof of the divine existing within the artist or a normal human expression devoid of any godlike connotations, it is perhaps the highest purpose to which we can strive. For the creatively intense person the relationship with creativity has already been established. Whether they have decided that they are creative or that they are not is not the defining category of the creatively intense. The fact that the internal conversation has been a profound one and that the resultant decision has been important to the concept of self is much more telling. There is an instinctive knowing of the importance of creativity.

Creativity is the cause of the world we know today. Every invention, every form of industry and technology, every social construct and every unifying belief system owes its origin to creative thought. This is the power of creativity. To be intensely creative is the greatest gift. It means that you are that much closer to the source of inspiration, that much more driven by imagination, and finally that much more capable of finding an ideal to shape the meaning and purpose of your life.

Creative intensity is not the same thing as artistic ability. Creative intensity is the drive to create. It expresses itself in a myriad of ways. The difference between a person who is creative and a person who is creatively intense is one of degree.

Imagine that the creative instinct, and I do believe that it's an instinct, is a little creature living inside your head. It may be blue and furry or sport multicolored feathers. Some of those little creativity creatures are tame. They sit nicely in the corner and come out when called. They cooperate well with the other little creatures in the brain and contribute here and there. Others of us have creativity creatures that are a little more hyper and vocal. They may interrupt in conversations, run amok in the middle of the night, or completely take over when the rest of the brain creatures have real work to do. They can be completely disruptive, a lot of fun, and at times brilliant. Those are the creatively intense creatures.

You may or may not have identified this intensity in yourself. You may have misinterpreted it as some undesirable trait like flightiness, inattention, anxiety, etc. What is certain is that as a person with one intensity, you are likely to have more. With creative intensity you are a little closer to your creature because it demands attention one way or another.

IMAGINATION

To those who have made the decision that they are not creative, I present proof to the contrary for your consideration. You may claim that it is simply an expanded definition of creativity. No matter, if it provides recognition of a natural talent that can be used to create within your life, it's worth contemplation.

Imagination is the key ingredient of creativity. We recognize imagination in children in part because they haven't been taught to be quiet about their imaginings. A child may have an imaginary friend who is usually to blame for any mishaps or stolen cookies. Or they may "see" fairies in the garden at twilight. These things are accepted in children to a degree, but at some point we begin to tell them that they must understand the difference between fantasy and reality. It becomes very important, and indeed it is. Joshua, the son of a very creative and intense friend, was less than two years old when he jumped from a second-floor balcony because he was sure he could fly. Don't worry; he wasn't hurt beyond a bruise or two.

His mother, however, was traumatized. Well-meaning parents always have and always will continue to downplay the role of fantasy in their children's lives.

As we become more adult we stop talking about the things we imagine until the imagination has been forced underground, but it doesn't stop. Particularly in intense people it never stops. It just stops talking out loud. Because we haven't given it attention, it is like a child left alone. It may continue in the beautiful fantasy world or it may go to a dark place. It seems that the imagination continues to try to explain the world even when we haven't paid it any attention. But it produces the explanation of a child. It isn't bound by reason, but by emotion. It is driven by fears and desires. If you think not, take a little time to check in with your imaginings. They are happening most of the time when we don't have to attend to what we're doing. That means that while we're driving, during lapses in conversation, walking down a hallway, taking a shower, or hosing down the patio, we have opportunities for the imagination to fill in the space. These things imagined are just barely within our awareness. You have to pay attention to catch them.

Today as I write I am in our little house in the mountains. Since it is so beautiful outside, I decide to do my meditation on the front deck in the sunshine. The sun feels warm and comforting after a cold night. There are the usual sounds of nature, birds chirping and insects buzzing past my head from time to time. In the distance I can hear the beep, beep of a truck backing up. It all blends into a song of sorts that make it through to my consciousness as I quiet my body and my mind. Overhead I hear what sounds like a small plane. And then it happens. My imagination has the plane dropping an engine. I picture it plummeting through the air headed straight for my tiny little head, which is in my imagination, blissfully unaware of the impending doom. I giggle a little and without looking up I go on with my meditation grateful for the example. This is exactly how the imagination plays when we aren't giving it any attention or purpose. These little imaginings happen in pictures that go past our awareness so quickly we usually miss them. Now that we're older they pretend to be about very adult things like danger from falling airplane engines. They play out scenes and pretend to warn us of danger. They pretend that we're someone else, or that we have what someone else has. They create relationships that aren't there. For the most part they pretend to be about real life with none of the limitations of normal life. There are no natural laws to obey, no limitations of time or space. We can be anywhere, any when. We can be in two places at once, flash into the future or live backward in time. We can change the outcome of an event by going back and living it differently.

Have you ever caught yourself running through a conversation you had recently and responding in a different way? It's a different quality than just saying, "I wish I'd said this instead." It's playing it out as if it really happened that way, complete with the reactions others would have had. You travel back in time and change the events to enjoy a different outcome. These imaginings are fighting to be heard and so with everything they can muster they appear to be adult. The childlike freedom to imagine and pretend has played the ultimate trick on us. It's pretending so hard to be an adult, concerned with very adult matters, that it has lost its playfulness.

Do you still think you don't have much of an imagination?

OVERACTIVE IMAGINATION

Then there are those who are certain of their imagination. They know it well because it is a constant companion. An active imagination can be great entertainment when you're stuck in a boring situation, but the very same imaginings can present a real problem when trying to go to sleep. My children, like most, had bad dreams when they were young. This is nothing more than the creativity creature running amok when the consciousness is asleep. But we can still guide it, even in our sleep. Years ago I heard a story about a tribe who put great value on dreams. It was an integral part of their culture. Each morning they would ask their children about their dreams and talk about them together. The expectation that dreams would be a topic of conversation every morning caused the conscious awareness to be more present in the dreams. As a result, lucid dreaming was common among this culture. Lucid dreaming is the ability to be completely aware during a dream state. As an aid to bringing awareness to the dream state, I instructed my children to remember to look at their hands. Whenever they could remember to look at their hands they were immediately conscious and in control. At that point, they could request help from anyone, and that person would appear to help. Then I told them that they could ask for anything they wanted. Even the bad guy in the dream would be forced to comply. They received all sorts of presents. It didn't take them long to start asking for things that could be taken into waking life such as poems.

An active imagination is standard equipment for the creatively intense. Just as bad dreams appear while the consciousness is sleeping, the imagination can cause all sorts of trouble in waking life when consciousness is not in control. Fear and anxiety fuel imaginings of every terrible possibility, which in turn further feed the fear and anxiety.

Our brains and bodies have a difficult time determining the differences between something imagined and something experienced. With an imagination running wild it's possible, even probable, that things imagined will have a very real impact on body and mind. There have been several studies on the effect that visualization of a physical action has on the body. In a study published in 1992, thirty college students were selected to perform internal imagery of exercise (imagining exercise), external imagery of exercise (video or other supplied images), or rest. Physiological responses were recorded in all three groups during imagined exercise, actual exercise, and rest. Not surprisingly both internal imagery and external imagery had some effect on respiration rate, blood pressure, and heart rate similar to regular exercise. While both methods had some physiological response, internal imagery was closest to actual exercise. This proves that what we imagine has a profound effect on our bodies, but what about the effect on mental states? A study published in 1997 in *Health Psychology* tested the effects of guided imagery and music on mood and cortisol (the stress hormone). They found that after six biweekly sessions, participants had significant decreases in pre- and postdepression, fatigue, and total mood disturbance as well as a significant decrease in cortisol. There should be no question now about the effect of imagination. What we imagine is very real to our bodies and minds.

INSPIRATION

Much like the imagination, inspiration seems to bubble up from nowhere. It is the spark and the thrill of creativity. Inspiration is the connection with the collective unconscious, with God, or with the universe, depending on your outlook. It is both the reason we hesitate to claim our creative nature and the reason we return to it with such passion and sometimes need.

Imagination without inspiration looks like the movies that run in our heads when we're not paying attention. It is full of rehashing current events in a different way or playing out fears. It is the little creativity that serves to remind us that it still exists. Our minds continue to volley for control. That control kills inspiration every time.

Inspiration is by definition out of control. It is wild. It behaves like a force of nature and, like nature, seems unpredictable. At times it is there, gracing us with ideas and visions, and then it's gone. The entire relationship between a mortal and inspiration has taken on the appearance of lovers. Artists have viewed inspiration as a woman, a muse, who can make their world full of life, abundance, and meaning. She can just as easily and for no apparent reason desert them, making life flat and full of frustration. This muse can't be forced, but must be invited, even seduced.

As the concept of inspiration develops here, you can begin to see how this is a love affair. Underdeveloped, it has the thrill, passion, and short life of infatuation. But a well-developed relationship with inspiration takes on the depth and closeness of mature love. It accepts us as we are. It is as much a friend as a lover. It is always there for us. And it is won the same way, with an awareness of what we can give instead of what we can take.

Inspiration is the seed for creativity. In order to have that seed produce its inherent promise, it requires hospitable conditions and nurturing. There is a quickening of the spirit during times of inspiration, but if the seed of that inspiration is to grow, it requires the ability and desire to carry it through long after the quickening has faded. It's easy to become addicted to the inspiration without the determination for following through. If you look in my closets or in my garage you'll see that I have a history of being a compulsive self-starter and a miserable self-finisher. There are unfinished projects to fill all the space I have. I absolutely love the beginning. The thrill of the inspiration can keep me from sleeping. I am obsessed until I can get my hands on the project. However, sometimes the determination I once felt to see the realization of the finished creation fades and fails me before the project is complete. It starts to feel like work, sometimes drudgery, until I finally put it aside.

The nurturing needed to manifest inspiration is like the work we put into building a mature, loving relationship. It's like the care and feeding we provide to our children or like the loving care we give to our parents as they approach the end of life. It's not always as exciting as the original creation of the idea. It is just what we do because we are who we are. It requires commitment; the bigger the creation, the longer and more demanding the commitment. As with all things, this is a choice.

I can look back on some of my unfinished projects and understand that they weren't that important to me. They were like a drug at the time, providing the high of inspiration without the commitment of completion. The fact that they sit unfinished in my closet or garage doesn't make any difference to anyone, me included. And the projects that enjoyed my continued energy and dedication are shining examples of what can happen when inspiration, imagination, and dedication meet.

Those unfinished projects sitting in my garage and closets and encroaching into the living room may not make a difference to me, but there is a risk to my relationship with inspiration with too many of them. As I start and fail to complete project after project, confidence in my ability to complete any creative act starts to wane. The repetitive "create, create, create," spoken by Pearl Buck in the quote at the start of the chapter is undoubtedly due to the thrill of inspiration. Another part of her quote gives a clue to the solution to the problem of unfinished projects. It has to do with meaning.

> . . . so that without the creating of music or poetry or books or buildings or something of meaning, his very breath is cut off from him.

When inspired to create something with very little meaning, the fortitude to complete the project is not long-lived. However the projects with meaning are almost always brought to fruition. And when they aren't, the creative urge continues. It haunts until it's satisfied.

CREATIVITY AS THERAPY

The need to create, when ignored, causes a sense of dis-ease. Mental and physical illnesses are a natural result of the creative urge pushed underground. Long have we recognized the link between creative genius and madness, but as much as we pontificate on the relationship, we haven't found an understanding. Van Gogh once said, "As a suffering creature, I cannot do without something greater than I—something that is my life—the power to create." Van Gogh may be the poster child for this pairing of creative genius and madness, but he has a lot of company. Einstein is thought to have suffered with Asperger's syndrome. Andy Warhol may have had autism.

Whether the dis-ease is a cause of creative genius or the creative genius is the cause of dis-ease can be debated, but the answer may not matter much. What we do know is that a creative act calms anxiety and helps to heal. My experience is that the greater my current involvement with creativity, the greater my sense of well-being. The American Art Therapy Association defines art therapy as

> a mental health profession that uses the creative process of
> art making to improve and enhance the physical, mental and
> emotional well-being of individuals of all ages. It is based on
> the belief that the creative process involved in artistic self-
> expression helps people to resolve conflicts and problems,
> develop interpersonal skills, manage behavior, reduce stress,
> increase self-esteem and self-awareness, and achieve insight.

Any sort of creative act has this healing power. It doesn't have to be a serious oil painting or a sculpture chiseled from marble. I have heard many stories of quilting, scrapbooking, singing, playing the piano, making a collage, and gardening providing a level of healing that wasn't available any other way. It is particularly useful for intense people who may have more sensitivity. If you are more likely to have been hurt, you are more likely to need this form of healing.

THOUGHT AS THE ULTIMATE
CREATIVE MEDIUM

We think of paints, clay, and paper as creative mediums. We also understand how lumber and building materials can be the mediums with which we create beautiful architecture. Stretch it further into words that can be used to craft stories, songs, or declarations that bring a new country together. There is something that each of these has in common, a medium that came before the clay or wood or paint. Each creation in the world begins as a creation in thought. Thought is the most versatile medium, with the capability to build a completed creation, erase it, and do it over again, and repeat that process dozens of times within a few minutes. This medium works so quickly you are often unaware of its creations. When you are aware of thought as the ultimate medium, you can begin to create in the realms of meaning, purpose, and idealism.

CREATING MEANING, PURPOSE,
AND IDEALS

Creativity is the method we use to explore and explain existence. It's the avenue to meaning and the founder of purpose in life.

On a fundamental level there is a need to explain nearly every event in our lives. If a tragic event occurs, perhaps the loss of a loved one, we need to find an explanation or meaning. Without that meaning the event will continue to haunt us. In the same way, we need to explain and provide meaning for much lesser events. A comment that hurts, a glance from a stranger, a choice someone else made that is different from a choice you might have made, really anything that occurs can trigger the meaning-making machine. That meaning-making machine is pure creativity. The same type of event will be used to create different meanings by different people. The resultant meanings create the flavor and tempo of life. That life may be happy or sad, aimless or purposeful, and any number of other variations all dependent on the meanings that are created and added to the internal map of reality.

Purpose is a type of meaning that is future-directed. Too often people see their purpose as some mystery. They think it is predetermined and that they have to go out and find it. Then they're never sure if what they found is real. Perhaps they misread some clue. Insanity! Purpose is a creation of your very own. It's as natural as any other creation, and it, too, starts with the medium of thought. The more pure and strong the thoughts used to create the purpose, the more pure and strong the purpose and its effect on your life.

An ideal is a refinement of meaning and purpose to a state of perfection. It is necessary to create an ideal as a signpost out in the future. It doesn't mean that the future will be that ideal, but it will always be standing there, marking the direction we should be going. The nature of an ideal is that it is unachievable. No matter how far you've come, the ideal seems to be just as far away. In this way the ideal is a perfect subject for the creative mind. It can be built with the only substance that can adequately represent it, thought.

The method of creating an ideal that will stand up over time and not lose its appeal is a little easier for the intense person. We favor big ideas and plans that some may consider grandiose and we are comfortable with the concept of perfection, as unachievable as it is. This ideal should be so big that it sounds impossible and so personal that it brings tears to your eyes when you think of it. Your mind is perfectly constructed to generate and hold ideals. The inspiration for an ideal is readily available to you if you've developed that long-term love affair with the muse.

An ideal is needed in order to focus for really big creative acts. One of the reasons that people fail with the law of attraction or attempts to manifest using any type of method is that they pick a goal instead of an ideal. A goal is something specific, measurable, achievable. A goal has to be concrete. And because of those limitations, it isn't big enough to hold your attention. If I have a goal of having a certain type of job, or owning a certain home, it may fit all the rules of constructing a goal, but it's going to get boring if I actually concentrate on it every day. Maybe the first thirty or sixty days will be all right, but after ninety or one hundred twenty days most people, and particularly intense and creative people, will be bored to tears with the whole idea. Goals are great for marking steps along the way. They can be used to measure progress toward an ideal, but they aren't strong enough to hold focus for really big creativity.

To develop creative intensity is not to become more creative. It is to know how to use the power of creativity, to be no longer at the mercy of the muse, but to have complete power over her with her consent. It is knowing how to hold an ideal and use it for focus and direction.

DREAMING TOO MUCH

Spending too much time with inspiration and imagination can be devastating and more than a little bit irritating to those around you. The result of such indulgence is a tendency toward procrastination, inability to be present, and sometimes a loss of connection to reality.

Imagination allows instant gratification. Imagine a project, and it's done just that quickly, without waiting and without work. If it doesn't turn out to your liking, it's just as simple to re-imagine it until you are very pleased. While this part of a creation is immensely satisfying, it really is only the first step. The trouble is that this step is so fun, and feels so creative, moving on to the next step can seem like reality slapping you in the face; it feels so much better to go on dreaming. But the price of that indulgence is the inability to actually create. In order to create, one has to balance imagination and action.

Another casualty of overindulgence in imagination is the ability to be present. Any time your imagination is entertaining you, you are not being in the present moment in the present place. This means that you are removed from the world, and from the people in it. That presents a problem if you spend too much time there. It creates distance from family and friends. It is like building a wall around yourself. There are times when that's a good response to a situation, but spending the majority of your time there is like a drug. It's just as addictive and it takes the same toll on relationships. Life is to be experienced.

Creativity is the essence of all life. It is the revelation of truth, beauty, and goodness. It is how we are able to conceive of our existence. It is our connection with each other and our method of understanding that connection. It is the only way we are able to find meaning and purpose in life. To develop our power of creativity there are three domains in which to practice. They are imagination, inspiration, and moving into action. For imagination, first we'll gain some control so that imagination doesn't control us, then we'll take a cue from Merlin and try living backward in time. For inspiration we'll learn how to seduce the muse. And for moving into action, we'll practice something that may sound counterintuitive. We'll learn the basics of planning and executing. The practices in the next chapter allow access to a level of creativity and a command over it that you never dreamed possible.

Important Points for the Impatient

- As we become more adult, we stop talking about the things we imagine until the imagination has been forced underground. But it doesn't stop. Particularly in intense people it never stops. It just stops talking out loud.

- Creative intensity is not the same thing as artistic ability. Creative intensity is the drive to create. The difference between a person who is creative and a person who is creatively intense is one of degree.

- Imagination is a key ingredient of creativity. The imagination that has gone underground is driven by fears and desires. It pokes its head out of the dark by presenting pictures that go past our awareness so quickly we usually miss them.

- Inspiration is the spark and the thrill of creativity . . . and it is addictive. Men have viewed inspiration as a woman, a muse, who can make their world full of life, abundance, and meaning. She can just as easily and for no apparent reason desert them, making life flat and full of frustration. This muse can't be forced, but must be invited, even seduced. The relationship with inspiration is like a love affair. Underdeveloped, it has the thrill, passion, and short life of infatuation. But a well-developed relationship with inspiration takes on the depth and closeness of mature love.

(continues)

(continued)

- Thought is the ultimate creative medium. Preceding literally every creation is that creation in thought. The inspired creative process has an added element of meaning, purpose, or an ideal. Using thought as the medium, the idealist creates what doesn't exist today. These dreams and ideals are at the root of every invention, new social structure, and medical or technical advance.

- The real difference between a dreamer and a creator is the ability to take ideas into the real world. This requires planning and action.

11

Creative Practices: Becoming a Creator

"There's no use trying," she said: "one can't *believe impossible things."*

"I daresay you haven't had much practice," said the Queen. "When I was your age, I always did it for half-an-hour a day. Why, sometimes I've believed as many as six impossible things before breakfast."

—Lewis Carroll, *Through the Looking Glass*

Imagine beginning a painting with no plan or vision, no message to convey, no model to interpret, and no idea of what you desire for the final creation. It may turn out to be one of those lucky accidents where the end product is very pleasing. The more likely outcome is a mess of paint on canvas. If your life were the canvas, imagination were the paint, and inspiration were the vision, would you be pleased with the painting? Do you have mastery over the paint? Does your vision thrill you?

Imagination is the medium with which we create our lives and inspiration, the reason. The practices in this chapter are designed to increase the skill and awareness you bring to the use of your imagination and to create a close personal relationship with inspiration such that the quality of your life will be transformed forever. It concludes with a very practical exercise designed to help make the leap from imagination and inspiration to true creation.

Practice 10

TAMING THE IMAGINATION CREATURE

Just as my children, and many others, have been able to exercise conscious control over their dreams, we can exercise conscious control over our imaginations in waking life. I haven't found a way to turn the imagination off; maybe because I've never looked for one. But I have found that I can have a direct impact on the types of things I allow my imagination to entertain. It starts with conscious awareness. Just as becoming conscious to induce lucid dreaming allows control over dreams, becoming conscious of imagination in waking life creates an opportunity to take control. An artist couldn't begin to create a masterpiece with paints and brushes that act on their own. In the same way, the creator in you can't begin until you have practiced control over the imagination. The ability to stop imagining unpleasant things has to come first.

1. Take preventative measures: Guard yourself against reinforcing fear-provoking subjects on television or the movies. Just as you wouldn't allow your child to watch a frightening movie, you should monitor your own input. There are some simple steps you can take to begin controlling the unpleasant aspects of being very imaginative while preserving your creative nature.

- Avoid violence on TV (that includes the news), particularly before bed.

- Avoid conversations with people who love to entertain conspiracy theories.

- Have a stockpile of pleasant thoughts to go to as needed.

- Before going to sleep, purposely think about something pleasant.

- If nightmares are a problem, keep a notepad next to your bed to begin lucid dreaming. Whenever you wake up during the night, write down your dreams. When you can remember, look at your hand in your dream to start lucid dreaming.

2. Be the witness: When your imagination has taken you to a bad place, start by practicing being in the witness state (see chapter 3). The witness can become aware of the visions and ideas that the imagination automatically presents.

3. Redirect the imagination: The most direct approach is simply to deliver a stern "Stop!" to yourself. It may seem as though you're stopping yourself constantly at first. Perhaps you will be. However, eventually the imagination will stop presenting the subjects that were causing you distress. I know that this seems too simple. There should be a very complicated process for controlling the imagination, but this is what works.

4. Offer your imagination an alternative: For two minutes take yourself to another reality. Imagine having accomplished a goal or having realized an ideal. Feel it; see yourself completely involved in it. Imagine the sensations and the emotions, and savor it for a minute or two.

Practice 11

LIVING BACKWARD AND
FORWARD IN TIME

LIVING BACKWARD IN TIME

Merlin the Magician was said to have lived backward in time. Merlin was able to remember the future but not the past. Every good-bye was meaningless, but hellos were tearful and impacted him greatly. For Merlin the first hello was the ending of what may have been a long and meaningful relationship. And the final farewell was the beginning. Since there was no memory of the experiences he had had with that person yet, he felt nothing. For Merlin, just as good-bye came before hello, the end of a life came before the birth. Every object appeared fully formed and ended by being created. When you think about it for any length of time, you'll begin to see that living backward in time isn't really that different at all. There are beginnings and endings to things. It wouldn't appear to Merlin that the result is coming before the action. It might seem that the result is the cause of the action. If you were able to see the result of something before the creation of that thing, you too would think of the result as the cause of the actions that create it.

Take an example of some big thing, like a spaceship, and follow it backward in time. The path that was taken to create it becomes evident. The step after the completed spaceship—remember, we're going backward here—would be the testing. Then you would see its assembly, then the design. There might be subcontractors who provide a part, and that part would move backward to the mining of those raw materials from the earth. There would be the approval process to move forward with the building of the spaceship, and there would be the idea of that particular spaceship. The final point would be the concept of space travel as a possibility. In every case, whether you are following a spaceship, a computer, a building, or any other creation of humans backward in time, there is a point when the thing is nothing more than a creative idea.

The point of this exercise is to experience the best of both worlds. It helps to live backward in time in order to see a creation fully formed, but that experience is only helpful if we live the rest of the experience going forward in time. Developing the dexterity to move forward and backward in time is the ideal. For example, if I want to create a business venture, it helps to see that business fully formed in my mind. The size of it, the employees, the buildings, the colors, the signage, the balance sheet and every other thing about this business should be crystal-clear in my mind. I can visualize that an article in a national newspaper about my business is the starting point. Then I move backward in time to the national expansion. The next stage might be the planning for the expansion and securing capital. The next previous stage would be the regional expansion. And the next stage would have been the local newspaper running an article on the phenomenal success of the flagship location. And so on until I am sitting on the beach and the idea for the business strikes me.

I may currently be anywhere along this continuum of creation. At this point, having seen the completed story of my business creation, I have no trouble seeing the next step forward. It's not hard at all, because I've already been there, done that. Some of the steps may turn out to be slightly different than my "memory" of the future. Some of the steps may be identical. Undoubtedly some of the steps will challenge me. I may have to stretch and do things that are well out of my comfort zone, but they aren't as difficult because I've done them before in my future.

If I can see a completed creation, and follow it backward in time to the original idea enough times, I begin to see the reverse pattern much more easily. I see how an idea is taken to fruition. And I see how my idea might be taken to fruition. Things begin to look much more possible.

1. Select a quiet and comfortable place to sit quietly. Close your eyes and relax your body and mind.

2. Think of a creation, something that is real, something that already exists. It can be something in your home, an object of interest for you, or anything else that is complex enough to occupy your mind for at least fifteen minutes. Start at the end with the completed creation and begin to move backward. Slowly and carefully identify each step of the process of its creation moving backward to see each previous step. Continue on with previous steps until you have arrived at the original creative idea.

This exercise should be repeated several times. The more often it's done, the easier it is to envision creation going forward in time.

LIVING FORWARD IN TIME

Everything that is external is an effect. Every external effect has a corresponding internal cause. We spend much of our time and energy trying to deal with and influence the world of effects. We mistakenly think that the "real" world is the external world and that is where we should focus in order to create. Our problems seem to come from the external world and it seems logical that the solution to those problems would be in taking action on the external. In reality the only place where we can create and cause anything is internal. By learning to focus on the internal, developing the power and control over our ability to cause, we have the ultimate power over the external world.

Nature has a way of creating that makes it look simple. A seed drops to the ground and, given a nurturing environment, begins a journey to become a plant. As the seed breaks open, a tentative root pushes through, seeking the dark moist earth below. The root, finding its place, sends out small shoots, which grow and dig deeper. A stem finally emerges and, pushing off the protection of the seed pod, breaks through the soil and reaches for the light. Leaves unfold. Branches spring forth and in perfect form support new leaves and finally the bud of a flower. Over time, the flower blooms and produces a new crop of seeds.

The beautiful simplicity of this creative act is an inspiration. The combination of persistence and fragility are stunning. While a root system will work around almost any obstacle in the ground, incorporating rocks and roots of other plants into its own support system, the plant can be easily destroyed by neglect or unsuitable conditions like a hot dry wind. Nature takes these setbacks in stride. If one plant dies, she's already working on many more. She employs flexibility and never-ending focus on a single ideal to ensure success.

A perfect accompaniment to the exercise of living backward in time is the practice of envisioning creation moving forward in time. This exercise can be alternated with the previous one as it pleases you.

1. Begin by taking the same position and go through the preliminary steps of relaxation.

2. Envision a seed. It can be any kind of seed to produce any plant you favor, a spring flower or an oak tree. In your mind's eye, place the seed in the ground. In this exercise you have the ability to see the growth underground, the roots pushing through the seed, and the determination with which the stem pushes off the seed to reach up and out. Watch and feel the

growth of each part as though it were a part of you. Feel the warmth as the first stem reaches for the sun. Continue to the full maturity of the plant. As you repeat this exercise you can choose different plants and experience a variety.

The combination of living forward and backward in time will make a shift in your consciousness. The relationship between cause and effect will be obvious to you, and you will begin to see creation as the most natural thing in the world.

Practice 12
SEDUCING THE MUSE

The muse, the source of inspiration, is living within you right now. It is your subconscious mind. Although it is a part of you, you may not be well acquainted. The relationship with the muse is perhaps the most misunderstood of all relationships. We think of inspiration as something outside of our control. It happens to us. It is apart from us and we have no expectation that we can command inspiration. We also have no understanding that we might have a responsibility to inspiration. If this were a relationship with a lover, it would be no wonder that she would leave.

How do you treat your lover? Do you listen when she talks? Do you make it a point to spend time together? Do you think of little ways to show love and devotion? Or do ignore her? Do you take her gifts and later throw them in the trash? Do you say you're too busy to spend time together and then fritter away your time in front of the television or computer?

Think of inspiration as a lover. This lover is special. This lover was made for you. The muse has no need or desire to go off and inspire someone else. You are the only one who matters. This is your personal muse. All she asks is that you spend time with her and listen to her ideas. She can be asked for grand ideas, little ideas, or next steps. It's as if she's been harboring all the dreams and interests and ideas that ever sparked in you, just waiting for this moment. She has the big and little ideas and is ready to share the next step in any creative process.

Not only does the muse have access to original ideas to share, but she also has access to a storehouse of information. If her home is in the subconscious mind, the vast stores of information collected throughout your lifetime that are beyond your waking awareness are the very fabric of her being. Her home is upholstered in your memories long forgotten. Her walls are papered with the knowledge you've been exposed to and never even noticed. The influence of all the people in your life, the wisdom shared with you when you were a child, the subjects memorized for the test and soon forgotten, and more are all there waiting for you simply for the asking.

This is not a relationship to be entered into lightly. The result of a flirtation with inspiration without the commitment of a relationship is bound to leave you feeling empty. The thrill of the romance only makes the eventual desertion that much more painful and the void depressing. Make no mistake that inspiration will leave you if you don't treat the relationship with respect and, yes, love.

The muse is fond of attention. She wants to be heard and appreciated. The more often you spend time with her, the more she gives. If her gifts are appreciated, she doubles her endowments. The following exercise is a recipe for beginning and nurturing a relationship with the muse. If followed regularly, a deep, meaningful bond is certain. The muse will become a faithful companion ready to put all her energy toward achieving your dreams.

The exercise is different than anything we've done so far. It isn't about putting information in, learning, or even growing. This exercise is about building a relationship through listening.

1. Before going to your usual quiet, comfortable sitting place, find a notebook and a pen. This notebook should be new, and it should be used solely for this purpose. Later, you can use the notebook to write your requests for the muse. For now, you will only record her first whispers in your ear. This is how she will know that you have decided to listen. She may approach the relationship tentatively and give only little bits at first, or she may blow you away with huge realizations and inspirations, the kind of thing that makes you slap your forehead and say, "Why didn't I see that before?"

2. Sit comfortably and close your eyes. Keep the notebook within reach. Relax your body until it's very still. Now still your mind. You can use a mantra such as "Om" or just concentrate on your breath. I use a visual mantra that appeared for me. I "see" a dark shape of an eye. It's perfectly symmetrical, and although it seems to move I try to keep it in the center.

3. Let the thoughts that take over roll past. When you notice them, just acknowledge them and move back to your mantra or point of internal focus. After some practice you may find that your conscious mind will allow the rest and go to a place where thoughts cease. This takes time. I've found that the muse is very active and loves to communicate so much that she doesn't have to wait for this opportunity. Still the communication is much better once you can get your conscious mind to back off for a while. This exercise can go on as long as you like. I find that twenty minutes is a natural amount of time for me. You will find your own time. Most people find anything from fifteen minutes to an hour feels right.

4. When the meeting with the muse is done, you may feel the need to write in the notebook. You may have had a thought you don't want to lose. These may be her first words to you

in a long time. Don't worry if nothing comes to you at first. Sometimes the communication comes through and doesn't make it all the way to consciousness. These little gems sneak up on you during the first hour or two after the exercise. Be sure to record them.

Most of the exercises in this book are designed to be done for a limited time. An intensity is developed and tuned by each one. This exercise, however, is designed to be done regularly forever. It gets to be more exciting and rewarding as time goes by. The insights and inspirations provided become a guiding light in your life, and you will grow to treasure them.

Practice 13
CREATIVITY IS IMAGINATION IN ACTION

Creation requires planning, prioritizing, and taking action. "Argh," I can hear the big sigh now. But planning and prioritizing don't have to be dull and without passion. This is one of those areas that would be taught in schools and supported by parents setting an example if intensity were the norm. Since nonintense people don't have the problem of getting lost in imagination, the path out of imagination and on to getting things done isn't normally taught. When intense people don't develop this skill, we run the risk of never bringing our best ideas to any kind of substantial completion.

It stands to reason that books on planning, prioritizing, and taking action to accomplish goals would be created by intense people who have finally found a solution to this common challenge. Alas, most of the books and systems are created by and for nonintense people and, as such, don't work for us intense people. I found one that came from a different starting point. It starts with finding what is important enough in your life, what you care deeply enough about, to want to create. Then it works with that passion to guide you through an incredibly simple and effective method to accomplish it. It was written by Steven Covey, who I've determined must be an intense person. The book is *First Things First*. This was one of those life-changing books for me. Not only did it help me to prioritize the actions I take in life, but it also filled in the gaps I have in being organized. Face it: Most intense people have trouble with organization. I'm not claiming that after reading a book I'm now an organized person; far from it. But I am completely capable of organizing the things I need to do for those areas most important to me. I can take imagination and inspiration through the planning and doing phases into creation. That's pretty powerful.

This may be the single most impactful exercise in this book. Read one of the great books on planning and moving into action, and implement the system. This one thing will change everything for you. You can move from being a dreamer to a being a creator. Here's a list of suggestions. One of them is sure to resonate with you.

First Things First by Steven Covey

Getting Things Done by David Allen

Zen to Done by Leo Babauta

Important Points for the Impatient

- Practice 10: Taming the Creativity Creature allows the imagination to stay intact but provides direction about which things you are willing to entertain and which are off-limits.

- Practice 11: Living Backward and Forward in Time begins developing the ability to recognize cause and effect as it appears in creative enterprises. Just like Merlin the Magician, the exercise will have you live backward in time, where good-byes are the beginning, hellos mark the end, and objects appear fully formed and disappear with their creation. The flip side of this is a complementary exercise of living forward in time. The two together provide a deep understanding of cause and effect.

- Practice 12: Seducing the Muse is the beginning of a life-long relationship with a part of you that will reliably produce insight, inspiration, and access to a vast store of information. This exercise will increase your capacity for living a full and rewarding life, no doubt about it.

- Practice 13: Creativity is Imagination in Action is the final step and perhaps the most important. Learning and employing a system that aids in taking ideas through planning and action results in the ability to truly be a creator.

12

Understanding Moods

A unicorn appeared one day
And flew me to the moon
The donkey brought supplies and love
And warned of waning soon
The lamb was there to comfort me
In softness like a womb
The tiger, I discovered then,
Was I, in full costume

—MARTHA BURGE

Emotional intensity is expressed in both moods and emotions. Emotions are an immediate response to a stimulus. By definition they arise spontaneously. Moods are sustained emotions that color the way we see the world and the way we act within it. Emotional intensity affects both. While moods may change temporarily throughout life, such as a long-term emotional state experienced in times of grief, the base mood with which we approach life has a certain unmistakable flavor that remains fairly constant.

Emotional intensity causes both moods and emotions to be felt more strongly, giving them a profound influence over us. The prolonged mood that influences so much of how we build and use our internal map of reality is referred to as a temperament. Some say we are born with it. Others say it creeps up on us when we aren't looking. The bottom line is that the mood we carry into each day has a direct effect on our experience of life. By understanding our own default moods, we can better understand why we do what we do and how to work best with our unique nature to bring about changes we desire in our lives.

UNDERSTANDING MOODS

Rafael Echeverria, one of the early contributors to the concept of ontological coaching, proposed an interesting model showing four basic moods in life. He suggested that we each have a default mood that we return to when event-based emotions are not leading us in any other direction. Those moods are based on our acceptance or rejection of either the way things are ("what is") or with what could be ("possibility").

Peace and Resentment

The moods of peace and resentment are related to the acceptance or rejection of the way things are. Included in the category of "the way things are" are past and current events. Resentment shows up as recurring topics. It has persistence. When a person continually returns to past events or focuses on situations they determine to be wrong or causing insult or injury, they are in the mood of resentment. The opposite mood is peace. Although the person living in peace may not like the way things are, there is a general acceptance of the world as it is.

Ambition and Resignation

The moods of ambition and resignation are related to the acceptance or rejection of possibility for the future. More specifically they are related to a person's view of their ability to effect change by taking action. Ambition refers to the propensity to take action. Action shows up in conversation (for action, not complaining), making changes, taking risks, and direct confrontation. The person predisposed to action will be the one you think of when something needs to change, the one who isn't afraid to take a different path. Resignation is the propensity not to take action. People who default to resignation may not take action even when change is desired. It's a state of surrender. In its extreme form, it is a state of hopelessness.

MOOD ANIMALS AND MAKING CHANGE NATURALLY

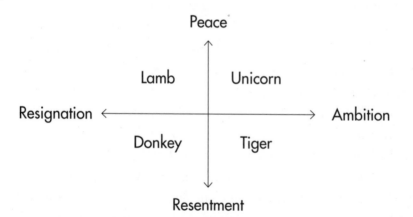

This chart represents my altered version of Echeverria's model based on the opinion that each of us has a relationship both to reality ("what is") and to possibility ("what can be"). Our real default mood has to take into account the combination. The vertical line represents your relationship to reality. To reject reality creates a mood of resentment. To accept reality creates a mood of peace. The horizontal line represents possibility. To reject possibility creates a mood of resignation. To accept possibility creates a mood of ambition. Using animals (lamb, donkey, tiger, unicorn) to symbolize each of the mood combinations helps with an intuitive understanding of the mood. Each mood animal falls into a quadrant on the chart. There isn't any one correct or best quadrant. Each has its positive and negative aspects. The point of this model is to help you understand your default mood. This is your nature, and one has to live according to one's nature. It also helps you understand the methods that may work best for you to bring about the changes you would like to see in your life. Each mood animal has a unique method of incorporating change.

The Lamb

Lambs represent people living in the combined moods of peace and resignation.

They are gentle and have a defining characteristic of giving comfort to others. The mood of peace contributes to the way they approach life by accepting not only the circumstances of life but also people as they are. Having experienced heartache of their own, they are incredibly compassionate to others in need. These are the people that others turn to when they need comfort.

The mood of resignation can cause lambs to feel unable to change circumstances around them, and the mood of peace flavors that resignation with a quiet creative instinct to create a better world, if only in fantasy. They are likely to have a well-developed imagination that can give rise to fascinating creative endeavors.

Being in a supportive environment allows them to blossom. When they do reveal themselves, their creativity and warmth draw people to them. They are strong contributors to their social groups.

Lambs can always be counted on to contribute to a bake sale, participate in a charity drive, or bring a warm meal to a person in need.

A big part of the lamb's nature is excitability. When secure, they are fun and lively. When insecure, they are anxious and fearful. The difference between security and insecurity is fragile for lambs. They are emotionally sensitive and easily wounded. The lamb would never consciously hurt another human being and so the thought that someone could hurt them is hard for the lamb to understand. While other mood animals may react to emotional blows by putting up defenses, the lamb doesn't. An emotional blow is fully felt and the wound is profound, resulting in sadness rather than anger.

Lambs are accepting of most change, although they don't naturally drive change in areas where they are uncertain. That's reasonable enough, but in order to make profound life changes, they have to take a more active role. Lambs are more likely to defer to someone else's judgment. This can be a good way to get started on a path of their choosing, but when giving that kind of authority to another person, they should carefully consider that person's true ability to guide them. Not everyone is worthy of their trust. Once they have found a mentor or decided on a path on their own, they need to build confidence. This is accomplished by taking action. It can be unnerving, but each small step builds confidence for the next. Small steps are the key, along with a source of support and encouragement.

The Donkey

Donkeys represents people living in the combined moods of resignation and resentment.

Donkeys are practical and realistic. Their demand for scientific proof (or other sources of ultimate authority) ensures that their beliefs and actions will produce the expected result. When anything new is presented, it's the donkeys who will ask for the proof, the credentials, and the peer review. Institutions that have withstood the tests of time and experience are their foundation. They place their trust in these institutions and enjoy being a part of them. When this well-considered trust is violated, the result is deep resentment.

Trust is an important theme for donkeys, not only with institutions, but also with people. The concept of the circle of trust has to have been created by a donkey. It conveys that a person is either in or out of the circle. There's no in between. If you're within the circle of trust, donkeys are kind, thoughtful, and caring companions. If you violate that trust, you're out, completely.

Similar to the circle of trust is the circle of influence. While the predominant mood of resignation prevails in much of the world for donkeys, they are capable of real ambition within their personal circle of influence. That circle may be at home, as a parent, in their work environment, or in a particular area of study. When empowered by the confidence they possess in that domain, they are capable of swift, decisive action. When faced with challenges outside of the circle of influence, they tend toward helplessness, which in turn creates frustration and sometimes anger.

Donkeys are hardworking, stable, and dependable. They are willing to put in long hours and enjoy being able to contribute by doing their part. You can count on them. They are predictable and dependable because that's the way they think the world should be. When the world doesn't cooperate with their high standards, they can become sarcastic, complain, or in extreme cases suffer from depression.

Donkeys aren't comfortable with change and don't see the point unless the process meets their high standard of proof. They are more agreeable to change when the path has already been put to the test. The path should be proven, the steps documented, the results nearly ensured. Still, life-altering changes are possible if desired. The current situation has to provide enough motivation to think about change.

The change has to be well-defined, having steps along the way and a clear destination point. It's best to allow some time to become familiar with each step, reducing the feeling of danger or discomfort by exploring the step in detail before taking action.

The Tiger

Tigers are the representation of the combined moods of resentment and ambition.

The presence of resentment makes tigers conscious of what is wrong in the world. This awareness of injustice, unfairness, and other perceived wrongs, combined with ambition, creates an irrepressible desire to take action. When the resentment is focused and the ambition well-thought-out, the result is an innovative leader. Most social reform leaders are tigers due to their ability to hold on to what's wrong and their belief in their ability, or rather, necessity, to do something about it. They are driven and intense. Very little would change without tigers. They are self-starters and idea generators. Their need to take action can result in very creative and innovative approaches to solving problems. They approach their work with a level of independence and free thought that reveal an entrepreneurial spirit. They are assertive, self-confident, and quick thinkers.

In relationships, tigers are both the greatest ally and the fiercest enemy. Since tigers are open and honest, there will be no doubt which side you're on. They are warm, caring, and generous to their "streak" (the proper name for a group of tigers). If you are in their group, you'll feel the backing of someone who would fight to the death on your behalf. They aggressively defend what they consider to be theirs, including their people. However if you present a threat, they are a formidable enemy. This is why tigers have retractable claws: Now you see them; now you don't.

Despite showing assertiveness that sometimes approaches aggressiveness on the outside, tigers are really very sensitive people. The tough exterior serves as a defense for a mushy interior. This is often misunderstood and is the secret to dealing with tigers. If you really understand how sensitive they are, and you respect that, you'll always be on the soft side of their hearts.

Tigers enjoy change, particularly change of their own design. The underlying mood of resentment provides plenty of opportunity to see what needs to be changed. Ambition provides the means to do so. The challenges for tigers are designing a change in one direction and more carefully selecting actions. With a plethora of things within conscious awareness in need of change, tigers can try to go in too many directions at once. Just as the power of a magnifying glass can focus the sun's rays to ignite a fire, it has little effect when the magnifying glass is constantly moving around. Or as the Pointed Man says in the film *The Point*, "A point in every direction is the same as no point at all."[30] When a tiger has chosen an area for change that is worth focusing on, the actions to be taken should be well considered. So anxious are tigers to make a move that they sometimes make the wrong move. The first action that comes to mind may be the best next action to take, or it may not be. Take your time, and choose wisely.

The Unicorn

Unicorns are the representation of the combined moods of peace and ambition.

It's no wonder why the unicorn represents this default combination of moods, as both are rare and awe-inspiring. Unicorns are so rare that I was convinced they didn't exist in adult form. I see this quality in children sometimes. My theory had been that these children will morph into a lamb, donkey, or tiger at some point, probably due to some emotional injury. And that may be the case. But I have now met one adult who is a natural unicorn, so I know they do exist. I also recognize that unicorns are re-created as adults when their emotional development has reached its peak.

The prevailing mood of peace makes unicorns easy to be with. They generate a sense of well-being that is subconsciously felt and appreciated by others. Their acceptance is palpable and generates a sense of ease. Even people who are likely to be self-conscious find themselves relaxed when with a unicorn.

The combination of accepting things as they are (peace) and feeling capable of generating change in positive directions (ambition) makes the experience of the world lighter for them. Although they are often very empathic, and sometimes actually feel the pain of others, they bring their natural joy to the situation. A sense of playfulness makes them not only comfortable to be around but fun, too.

The unicorn is completely comfortable with being in the lead. They can plan and take action to effect change with ease. Since the underlying mood doesn't provide staying power in their convictions, as resentment does for tigers and donkeys, they must develop a strong sense of conviction in order to be effective leaders. Without that, they tend to tire of their direction when they lose interest.

Unicorns are still subject to emotions. Peace and ambition are the default moods, but events still cause emotional reactions. Unicorns are as likely as any other to be sad or angry, but they seem to be more resilient.

Unicorns are also very comfortable with change. The unicorns who have been re-created as unicorns in adulthood are already proficient in change. Natural unicorns are, like children, very capable of change, but not always able to maintain focus in one direction. Because resentment is absent, it can't be used to provide the staying power for a direction for change. Motivation has to be found elsewhere. Developing a deep conviction, a purpose worth your time and energy, and something that is big enough to continue to interest you is the solution.

■ ■ ■

The fun in this model is in classifying all your friends and family. Everyone I know who has been exposed to this heads out on a tangent to find the mood animal for each person in their life. It makes great conversation and actually provides some insight into behavior. I'll caution you: People don't fit neatly into categories and are seldom in only one category; they just have leanings one way or another.

The value in this model is an opportunity to stop and consider your nature. When designing change in your life, going against your nature is never a good idea. The power you'll gain from going with your nature will make a difference in becoming the person you wish to be, doing the things you want to do and having the success you desire.

Important Points for the Impatient

- We all have a default mood or disposition that has a dramatic effect on every aspect of life. These default moods are the result of our relationships with both reality and possibility. Having the tendency to either reject or accept reality and possibility give us some combination of peace, resentment, resignation, and ambition.

- Each possible combination of the above moods is represented by an animal. Unicorns, donkeys, tigers, and lambs are representations of both a disposition and the method to best approach change.

- The model is not only fun, providing a model to analyze friends and family, but also practical, giving a prescribed best method of effecting change in your life by going according to your nature instead of fighting it.

13

Emotional Intensity

There is no coming to consciousness without pain.

—C. G. JUNG

Intensity belies the sensitivity in our souls. We are the bewildering combination of fragility and exuberance. We are sensitive and easily hurt, and at the same time we come on too strong, sometimes striking fear in others. The emotional highs and lows are difficult to contain. The amount of energy expended to appear "normal" can exhaust and discourage us. But the highs are too wonderful for words, making it all seem worthwhile again. Because we seem to have little control over whether we are experiencing the glorious highs of positive emotions or the dreadful lows of negative emotions, life can feel like a wild ride. But given that emotions are the only thing that creates drive, I'll take them full strength, thank you. Through understanding the nature of intense feelings, there is an opportunity to change our world from the inside out. Negative or unpleasant emotions, once understood, become a tool for self-understanding and growth. That growth leads to a new level of peace and happiness never before imagined. Instead of intense feelings being a curse, they are allies in becoming the person we wish to be.

THE INNER EXPERIENCE OF
EMOTIONAL INTENSITY

Because emotional intensity, like all intensities, is a matter of degree, we don't always know that our experience of the world, particularly the emotions we feel, are more intense than those felt by others. Sometimes the only way we recognize that our emotional lives are fuller and more extreme is by the labels others put on us. This particular intensity makes others uncomfortable, and so the labels are not very nice. Drama queen, crybaby, and hothead are tame compared to the disorders piled on some by well-meaning psychologists and psychiatrists such as anxiety disorder, mood disorder, bipolar, and other forms of psychoneurosis.

Even when we're experiencing good emotions, our intensity can intimidate others. The very presence of strong emotions can be perceived by others as a threat or deemed to be a lack of self-control or a lack of maturity. I used to buy into that story. I believed that others experienced emotions as strongly as I did and simply had remarkable self-control. But the self-control theory didn't pan out. I realized that they are expressing the emotions they feel in exactly the amount they feel them. They are not masters of self-control. They have less intense emotions.

And so the primary internal sensation of emotional intensity is one of insecurity and guardedness. We become aware of the fact that to be completely relaxed, to be one's self, results in negative responses from all but our closest friends and family who are more accustomed to us. To be too happy, too excited, or too upset—especially too upset—makes others uncomfortable. They see us as out of control, so we learn to guard ourselves.

Feelings of insecurity stem from the reactions of others to the natural expression of emotions. Themes of feeling socially awkward or avoidant may surface. Many of us are introverts, only feeling at ease and able to regenerate energy while alone or with a few trusted friends. Being around anyone else requires energy to be on guard.

Another aspect of being emotionally intense is emotional sensitivity. Just as sensory intensity creates an enhanced experience of the five senses, emotional intensity creates an enhanced experience of emotions. This can leave a person vulnerable to emotional wounding. A situation that would have been ignored by less sensitive people can devastate a more sensitive person.

We know that children who were raised in uncertain environments, such as having a primary caregiver with abusive tendencies, pay closer attention to emotional cues. Regardless of what the caregiver is saying, their very survival depends on being able to read behind the words. A slight change in tone or a minuscule muscle movement provides more accurate cues about the state of mind of the caregiver than their actions or words. In much the same way, emotional sensitivity creates an environment where the benefit of being able to read the emotional cues of others is needed to avoid emotional pain. When a person is saying something that doesn't match their emotional state, the emotionally sensitive person can detect the inauthenticity. For some, this sensitivity translates into being able to feel the emotional climate in a room or emanating from another person. It may seem to be so thick that one assumes everyone can feel it. We not only can easily sense the emotional climate but also are much more deeply affected by it. Living with someone who is depressed can cause a mirrored depression in the intense person. Because of this, most of us can remember being drawn to those who are happy and seem carefree.

Emotional intensity leads to learning and complexity. Let me explain. There are different methods of learning. Some things in life are learned by repetition; others are modeled by someone and we learn by watching. Psychologists have known for years that the most effective way of learning something is to combine information with an emotion. This is particularly true for an intense person. The presence of pain, pleasure, fear, or any other strong emotion first stores that information in the map, then carries the information immediately past the gatekeeper into the conscious mind. This is a natural human survival mechanism. If something is threatening, our neurological systems are preprogrammed to keep that information handy. If something is pleasurable, we are also preprogrammed to store that information for future use. Because we experience emotions more intensely, throughout life we encounter situations that cause us to store information more often than less emotionally intense people, and thus we become more complex. As additional information is stored, our personalities become more and more complex. We are capable of holding seemingly opposing opinions and characteristics within a cohesive whole. While it takes well into adulthood for us to begin to understand our own complexity, imagine how difficult it is for others to understand us.

THE OUTWARD EXPRESSION OF EMOTIONAL INTENSITY

Emotionally intense people are a minority of the population. It's estimated that 15 to 20 percent of people are intense, and not all intense people have emotional intensity as a primary expression of intensity. We begin to search for reasons why we are so different and why we suffer so much. A natural conclusion is that there must be something wrong. If consulting a psychologist or psychiatrist, the result will be a diagnosis. I sometimes wonder if psychiatrists are paid by the diagnosis, so happy are they to attach labels of disorder. Regardless of the motives, many emotionally intense people receive diagnoses of mental disorders. "Psychoneurosis" is a term that was used to identify any sort of mental or emotional disorder that could not be attributed to a neurological or organic dysfunction. It was considered to be a mild form of mental illness. The term is no longer in general use, but it is a useful concept to classify the types of mental disorders commonly attributed to intense people going through a positive growth process. As anxiety and emotional intensity do their work to drive us toward continued development, we are often viewed to have these types of mental disorders. They include mood disorders, anxiety disorders, emotional outbreaks, hysteria, any type of maladjustment and virtually any disorder that falls short of total insanity.

Treatment options for these "disorders," which may be nothing more than intensity, are medication and therapy. If you've been down this road, you have probably found the treatment to be less than ideal. Years can be spent on a path that cannot provide much help because the underlying condition isn't understood. If intensity is treated like a mental disorder, the outcome is a sensitive person who now believes herself to be disordered. Instead of understanding and taking advantage of the growth possibilities this condition affords, she changes her self-image to fit that of a person with a disorder.

Emotional turmoil doesn't have to be conquered alone. Therapists and coaches, familiar with Dabrowski's work, can help. Understanding the source of the emotional discomfort and the path leading to emotional maturity and peace of mind creates a new context. Dabrowski believed that the role of therapy was to provide a context for a person to understand and help himself. While traditional therapy views emotional crisis as something to be overcome to eventually return to a more stable state, Dabrowski proposed a positive view of emotional crisis and suffering as the dis-ease that causes the old view of reality to "disintegrate," leading to "re-integration" at a higher level.[31] This is the map falling apart and being rebuilt into a more productive form.

Many emotionally intense people have escaped the psychological labels, but none will escape the judgment of being out of the ordinary. Whether we are deemed too sensitive or edgy, anxious or thin-skinned, the differences are noticed. One of the problems for others is that we are difficult to predict emotionally. There seems to be no way to guess the situations that will evoke a strong emotional reaction. To an outsider it appears that we overreact to things and that there's no telling what may set us off. Since we are so complex, the ability for others to intuitively anticipate our emotional response to an experience is lacking. Our emotional reactions take even us by surprise sometimes. It takes decades to begin to understand your own complexity. While less complex people may understand themselves by their early twenties, we have a lot more to understand—exponentially more.

Throughout life the continual experience of intense emotions causes us to learn more about our emotional selves. We learn to anticipate those situations that may cause us to behave in socially unacceptable ways and avoid them if possible. This need to learn about ourselves, our reactions, and our expressions, while tiresome, is an opportunity for advanced development not afforded an average person.

DABROWSKI'S THEORY OF EMOTIONAL DEVELOPMENT

Kazimierz Dabrowski is best known for his theory of positive disintegration, also known as the theory of emotional development. It describes a process we follow as we grow emotionally. In his theory he describes the levels of development as more global states. It begins to sound as if we go from one level to the next as a whole. In reality it doesn't work that way. We grow a piece at a time. While our overall development can be categorized as being at one level or another, some parts of our inner selves advance before other parts. There may be times in life when we go through growth spurts, times when we aren't growing at all, and most often, times when we are going through small advances we hardly notice. The overall effect of these advances is an ability to handle situations in life with fewer negative emotional responses, more opportunities for positive or pleasurable emotions, and better relationships with ourselves and others.

This growth occurs as a result of problems. It is heightened by intensity, because our problems often become PROBLEMS. Dabrowski claims that only the intense individual is capable of reaching advanced levels of development precisely because of the turmoil created by being emotionally intense. He also includes intellectual and creative intensities in the prerequisites.

Looking at Dabrowski's theory through the lens of the internal map of reality makes the concepts a little easier to understand. When something is encountered that isn't well represented on our internal map of reality, it causes an internal crisis. Those who were blessed by circumstance with a robust map of reality don't encounter much in the way of crisis. They are the ones we refer to as well-adjusted. However most of us have maps that are insufficient to take us through life without incident. The feeling of crisis is the internal map of reality falling apart. Because we believe the map to be reality, it feels as if we, rather than the map, are falling apart. In Ontological Coaching this disintegration is called a breakdown. Indeed something is breaking down. The inner map is breaking apart, and what happens next can mean the difference between growth, stagnation, or mental illness.

When the map has been loosened, there is an opening to reform the map in a way that allows the current breakdown to dissolve. This is a restructuring of the map producing growth. Dabrowski called this process "positive disintegration." Disintegration is the loosening of the map. It's positive because it holds the possibility for growth.

Dabrowski identifies five levels of emotional development in his theory as follows:

Level 1

We start from a place where our internal map of reality is working for us. We are going through our day-to-day life without much of a problem. Dabrowski indicates that the majority of the population exists in level 1. While without much strife, it is also without much depth. The peace that many people find in level 1 isn't available for emotionally intense people. I'm sorry, but that's the truth of the situation. We will never be peaceful and content on the first level because, for us, the world has to cooperate, and it just doesn't. As sorry as that truth is, there is light at the end. Emotionally intense people have the capacity to go further. Not despite our emotional intensity, but because of it, we have the chance of reaching level 5, which is so rare and so satisfying. It is our only path to peace and happiness. It can take a lifetime, or it can happen much more quickly. The length and hardship of the journey is directly related to the amount of resistance we have to the changes along the way.

Level 2

Level 1 is broken when something occurs that creates an emotional problem. We call this a breakdown. Breakdowns come in all sizes, from continual nuisances to catastrophic conflicts. This is Dabrowski's level 2. He indicates that while many people find themselves in level 2, they usually drop back to level 1 after the situation has rectified itself in some way. At this level we seem to be at odds with the world. Because troubles are seen as being produced by outside events, the solutions are obviously to change the outside circumstances. This is normally not an easy undertaking.

The original structure of the map is the default stance on everything. If it is a map that allows for most circumstances we encounter in the world, then we have very little conflict and appear to be well-adjusted. If not, life appears to be fraught with problems and frustrations. Problems are evaluated on a pros and cons basis. We attempt to "figure it out." When figuring it out doesn't help, we may try methods to relieve the suffering, which sometimes leads to numbing the pain with drugs or alcohol. Attempts to alleviate suffering in this level are all within the domain of doing. We try to do different things to get different results. Unfortunately, there are a limited number of actions available based on the inner makeup of the person. What is possible for one person to do, another cannot even imagine. It is a changing of external events that causes the shift to level 2, and it is a change of external events that causes the return to level 1. If the map of reality is held too rigidly, or if the person lacks sufficient intensity, the map will take its previous form and nothing will have changed. The same kind of situation can cause the same breakdown over and over again without end because the map hasn't grown to handle it.

Level 3

Dabrowski identified level 3 as when one restructures the map to handle a breakdown instead of waiting for or trying to cause the external circumstances to change. When we become aware of the possibility of changing the map of reality to alleviate suffering, we also gain the first glimmer of the possibility of a better life. All kinds of things come into focus now. Instead of being thrown by circumstance, we realize that there may be another way. The turmoil we experienced in the previous level between ourselves and the outside world now turns inward. The parts of the outside world that have invaded our internal map of reality without question are beginning to be identified as not our own. In level 3 we begin to form our own opinions. We have to go through a reevaluation of the values and beliefs that were handed to us since birth. Chief among the concepts we question is our concept of self. This is the turning point. We start to form both a picture of a more ideal self and a willingness to go through some uncomfortable steps to strive toward that ideal.

The amount of resistance to giving up long-held attitudes, values, and beliefs is directly proportional to the amount of inner conflict experienced at this level. This is the map falling apart, allowing space for a new map to be built. Since we believe the map to be reality, it may feel as if the world is falling apart or, worse, that we are falling apart. That feeling causes us to resist. If we resist allowing the old map to fall apart, we are destined to suffer. If we allow the breakdown (or disintegration, or map falling apart) and watch it go, a new map will build that has a better understanding of the circumstances that brought about the crisis in the first place.

As changes begin to occur, there is a feeling of power. If our experience of the world is created more by our inner self than by the circumstances around us, we realize that we possess some level of control over how we feel. We don't have to be at the mercy of our emotions caused by events outside our control any more. Instead of evaluating based on pros and cons, we begin to evaluate based on higher and lower. We see that the explanations we held about the world and our place in it are not as concrete as we once thought. There are different explanations of a higher nature. Instead of a flat interpretation of the world and of ourselves, we sense that there are purposes and higher goals that are possible. We can now see that the new map, the new meaning we found, requires a more ideal self. We evaluate our inner world based on which meanings are higher, or more in tune with our ideal selves. Even in this level some parts of our internal maps are held more rigidly than others. Those parts may take bigger or repeated breakdowns before the map changes.

Level 4

After challenging our map on several parts of the terrain, and continuing to build a stronger and more inclusive map of reality, we may reach what Dabrowski calls level 4. At this point we have determined that the process works, and we more eagerly search for breakdowns, knowing the growth and eventual increase in positive emotions that are the result. We call this "declaring a breakdown." It is a voluntary process not brought on by external events at this point. This is a time of rapid growth. We begin to reap the rewards of our efforts in the form of advanced emotional development. There are fewer upsets and a noticeable increase in positive feelings. There is also a noticeable reduction of anxiety and dread. It takes more to cause a breakdown, and when they do occur, we are able to recognize them for the opportunities they are. As we work through the domains of our life and reach our ideals in one area or another, that portion of life is at peace. Our emotions are an ally in this process. Wherever there is discomfort, there is an area ripe for introspection and growth. A person can create a breakdown in any area in which growth is desired. This means that we decide that a particular area of the internal map of reality is not working as well as we would like. It may not be causing great discomfort, but we recognize that it's time to address some old parts of the map.

Level 5

Dabrowski's level 5 is a complete return to working with an internal map that handles the world. It is characterized by feelings of both peace and power. This is the hidden domain of lightness. At this level we are still emotionally intense. That will never change. There will still be pain. Loss of a loved one still produces grief. Some forms of suffering are inescapable as human beings. The difference is that we experience more positive emotions and become much more resilient. Resiliency allows a quick recovery from negative emotions.

■ ■ ■

In order to pass through these levels, intensity is a tremendous asset. The emotionally intense person has an opportunity to experience the conflict sooner in life than a nonintense person and to a degree that will spur on growth. Dr. Dabrowski contends that people who possess emotional intensity are the only ones who even have the possibility of this type of growth. I'm not sure that it's a prerequisite, but I know it helps. In addition to emotional intensity, a few other things are required. Extreme anxiety has to be eliminated. This was addressed in practices 1 and 2. In order to go down this path, where every fundamental belief and value is questioned, we have to have at least a moderate level of security, a feeling of being safe in the world. Next, we have to be willing to free ourselves from the attitudes, values, and beliefs that found their way into the internal map of reality when we weren't looking. Our family, friends, and society at large have implanted ideas that we accepted without question when we were very young. This unquestioning acceptance of ideas continues to a lesser degree as adults. We have to be willing to question now. In the questioning, we must determine what to keep, what to throw away, and what to create anew. We must be strong enough to go through the stress and the powerful emotional upheaval and develop the capacity to withstand ambiguity for a time. Finally, our sense of achievement must be developed as an internal mechanism and not depend on external rewards or acclaim.

CARTOGRAPHY: BECOMING A MASTER MAPMAKER

The description thus far of the experience of emotional intensity has been somewhat academic. The actual experience is anything but academic. Intense feelings can cause a level of suffering that most can't understand. Feeling wounded in a relationship or because of a loss is bad enough, but adding to that the feeling that you are too different, that you can't possibly be understood, creates a level of separation that is nearly intolerable. This sensation of being a stranger in a strange land is the one that drives many intense people to acts of desperation. The internal map of reality at this point looks something like this:

I don't fit in anywhere. There must be something wrong with me. Life feels like almost constant suffering punctuated by times of meaninglessness. It's just too much effort. Why am I here? What's the point?

Does any of this sound familiar? Let's break down the map into parts and see how it could be altered.

Map: I don't fit in anywhere. There must be something wrong with me.

- Alternate map: I'm intense. I know that we are in a minority of the population and it sometimes feels as if I'm alone. In reality about 15 to 20 percent of the population shares the trait of intensity.

Map: Life feels like almost constant suffering, punctuated by times of meaninglessness.

- Alternate map: I feel emotions more than most people, and when I suffer I do it big. It's all a part of being emotionally intense. In addition to being emotionally intense, I have a desire for meaning and purpose in life. Yeah, I'm deep.

Map: It's just too much effort. Why am I here? What's the point?

- Alternate map: In reality I am the only one that chooses what I do and why. I didn't see that before. I felt like a leaf blowing in the wind, and it was a cruel wind. Now I know that I'm not the leaf; I'm the wind.

It is widely recognized that mapmaking is both a science and an art. The reason that some geographic maps are better than others is because the cartographer represented reality in a way that provides useful generalizations, accuracy, and an aesthetic value. These maps work to navigate reality and enhance the experience at the same time.

Our internal map of reality, which contains our interpretations and generalizations and provides all the meaning in life, may or may not be accurate and enhance our experience of life. Whether our internal map of reality is one that produces pleasant or unpleasant results is entirely a matter of chance. This may be good news, in that you aren't responsible for your circumstances, but the better news is that you can remake your internal map of reality. Adjustments to the map allow a different experience of reality. It seems as if the world is changing.

The internal map is made up mostly of meanings. Every experience we have is interpreted by the gatekeeper. We aren't consciously aware of the decision process to allow information in or discard it. Once it is allowed in, it is interpreted by our internal map. This is where we assign a meaning to the event. For example, if a car cuts us off on the road, an event has occurred. That event will be interpreted by different people in different ways, causing different emotional reactions. One person may think that the driver of the other car is a jerk and that the act of cutting them off was an intentional act of violence, akin to pulling a weapon. Another person may think that the driver has too much on their mind and isn't paying attention. Still another may think that they narrowly escaped an accident and feel grateful to be safe. One of these interpretations is as accurate as the next, given that we don't know what the other driver was thinking. Why does each person have a different interpretation? They have different maps. Each map assigned a different meaning to the same event. Each meaning predisposes them to different emotional states. Instead of going through life being controlled by a map, which you didn't create, you can choose to change the map.

The challenge in becoming a master mapmaker is in the ability to let go of the old map. Much of the old map was created to keep us safe. The more the meanings in the old map are tied to safety, the harder it is to let them go. For those who experienced difficult, unsafe, or traumatic childhoods, there are parts of the map that are held rigidly. Even as adults, traumatic experiences create rigid areas of the internal map. The more rigidly the map is held, the more suffering will be encountered, both before and during the process of rebuilding the map. With the old map, suffering is experienced every time the map doesn't accurately represent reality. If my map has a territory for how an employer is supposed to treat employees, and that doesn't match with how my manager is treating me, I suffer. I can try to change my manager, but that isn't very likely to have much effect. Instead, I can rebuild that portion of my map to include people in positions of power who don't behave as I believe I would in the same position. There is now a territory in my map called "less-than-adequate managers." It doesn't have to cause me emotional strife. It just is.

There are also conflicts built right into the old map. Most original maps contain conflicting information. If a map contains the two conflicting ideas, everything seems to be all right until they run into each other. For example, Susan believes that education is very important. She spent years as a teacher and believes in her heart that education is a foundation for a better future. She also has strong opinions about how a grandmother is to behave. She's proud that she has kept the perfect balance between being a part of her grandchildren's lives without interfering in their parents' role as parents. Now the two beliefs are colliding. Her grandson has announced that he's decided not to attend college, and her daughter is supporting his decision. Does Susan interfere? Is it more important to convince her grandson that college is the best direction, or is it more important not to interfere with her daughter's parenting? Conflict!

Once you understand that the map is just a map, you're free to start the redesign process. That's easier said than done. A basic concept that helps loosen the grip of the old map is that nothing, and I really mean nothing, has any intrinsic meaning. Things are only things; they don't mean anything other than the meanings we give them. People are only people. The meanings we put on people and our interactions with them are from our map and nowhere else. No situation, interaction, person, place, or thing has any meaning other than made-up meanings we assign to them. Oh, I'll bet you've got something in mind to challenge me on this, right? If your example holds an intrinsic meaning, then it will mean the exact same thing to every person on earth, for all time. It doesn't seem so intrinsic now, does it? I realize that this can be a disturbing thought. If the meanings by which you lead your life aren't real, then what does it all mean? Is there nothing of true meaning? Isn't that a dismal outlook? On the contrary, it's an outlook that is full of possibility.

In this journey of discovery and creation of new maps, our emotions are a priceless tool. The only way to find the areas of the map that aren't serving us is by listening to our emotions. The upset caused by a map that doesn't match reality or the discrepancy between our current and ideal selves is the key. Our strong emotions are the reason we can progress. They create the drive. Emotional intensity not only makes it hard to ignore the problem areas, but also prepares us for the process of mapmaking. We've been through a lot and that gives us the strength needed to rebuild a world. That's exactly what this is: rebuilding your world from the inside out.

Important Points for the Impatient

- Emotions are the only way that any human being creates the drive to accomplish anything. Because our emotions are so strong, we have the gift of a strong drive that can be used in the process of emotional development.

- It is possible to reach an uncommon level of happiness and peace through a process outlined by Dr. Kazimierz Dabrowski. Throughout the steps of emotional growth, our negative emotions act as the catalyst to question and ultimately rebuild our view of reality, our self-image, and our value systems, resulting in a cohesive new self.

- The result of this process is an enlightened state where we are living in peace and harmony. Happiness naturally bubbles up, and negative emotions, while still present at times, are less frequent. We find ourselves to be resilient.

14

Emotional Practices: Emotional Growth and Power

When we are no longer able to change a situation . . . we are challenged to change ourselves.
—Viktor E. Frankl, *The Unheard Cry for Meaning*

Emotional development is much more important for the emotionally intense person. It makes the difference in every aspect of life. Without developing this intensity, we are thrown to the emotions caused by situations in our lives as if we have no control. It doesn't have to be this way.

As the center of control moves from outside of yourself to inside, you no longer need to be thrown to a way of feeling. You don't have to be that leaf blowing in the wind. You can create your own emotional field and with it your own drive. I also want you to know that these intense emotions, these complex and troublesome times, are not without purpose. The suffering you've endured in this life is purposeful. It has endowed you with a unique capacity you've yet to fully understand.

Our dreams are both created and fueled by emotions. By understanding your intensity and practicing the exercises presented here, you will find that emotional intensity can be the greatest gift of all. It can fill your life with warmth, close rewarding relationships, tenderness, excitement, and a drive that makes the difference between just getting by and being wildly successful.

There are three practices offered here to aid in your journey. They are offered with personal insight into the value they add. Along with the practice of these concepts, I hope to be able to provide a context for your struggles and achievements along the way. This is a brave person's path. Not many will attempt it, and indeed, not many are suited for it. As an emotionally intense person, you are already equipped with the primary component required. This is what Dabrowski called the third element. He recognized that there are both nature and nurture elements (heredity and environment) that control our ability for advanced development. But he also found a third element. This third element is exactly what I have been describing throughout this book: intensity.

Mapmaking is explained on three levels, one for each of the levels of emotional growth. The one you choose to concentrate on will depend on the type of breakdown you are experiencing. As you move from level 2 through level 3 and on to level 4, a different concept of the map is useful. In level 2, the map is constructed to provide a more accurate representation of reality. In level 3, it breaks down entirely, creating a void to be filled in a very personal and creative way. In level 4, the map is refined and the self is adjusted to better fit the ideals and values instilled into the map.

Quiet contemplation and meditation are useful throughout the process. Each type of meditation, concentration, and contemplation proposed though this book provide the quiet and focus needed here. By now, if you've been trying the practices in each chapter, you've begun to notice some changes in yourself.

Practice 14
MAPMAKING AT LEVEL 2

You believe the things you believe because, in your experience, they're true. But remember, the gatekeeper only lets information in that is either supportive of your view, interesting, or dangerous. Any events in reality that don't fit your ready-formed view of reality will not make it past the gatekeeper unless you find them interesting or they present a threat. There could be a plentitude of evidence that contradicts your view of the world that goes without notice. This mechanism serves to continually reinforce your current view, your map of reality. It proves over and over again that your map is accurate, whether it is or not.

At level 2, breakdowns are experienced as problems that exist "out there." Each breakdown signifies a loosening of the map in an area that isn't working. Each person has a strict set of expectations for the way people should behave and the way events should transpire. When things don't go as expected, the map tells you that something isn't right. It creates turmoil. Each time this happens, there's an opportunity to compare the map to reality. Where the map doesn't match reality, the map can be altered. Changes to the inner map at level 2 are relatively straightforward. In any conflict, simply identify reality and the corresponding area of the map causing the turmoil for you.

Example:

Reality: There is a person at work who is not completing their assignments on time and having a negative impact on our mutual project. The things I have tried to change his approach to the project haven't had an effect.

Internal Map: People should take their work seriously. They should be conscientious and take pride in the work they produce. It is the least they can do as a part of the team. To do otherwise is not only irresponsible but also damaging to everyone associated with the project.

Mismatch: Look for the "should," "shouldn't," "always," and "never." People *should* take their work seriously . . . That's the map. "Should" doesn't exist in reality. In reality, some people don't take their work seriously.

New entry to the map: Some people don't take their work as seriously as I do. It will sometimes cause projects to fail. It does not have to cause me to be upset. It just is. Whether I am upset or calm, I can still take actions regarding the situation. In fact, I may have a clearer head and take more effective action if I am not upset. No amount of upset is going to make all the people in the world or even all those in my environment care more about their work.

■ ■ ■

Throughout level 2 it's possible to reevaluate your internal map, make an adjustment, and relieve the tension and turmoil, although we can't always plan how the new element of the map will be created. In any level 2 breakdown, there is a triggering event.

1. The first question to ask yourself is, "What is reality in this situation?" It helps to write it out. Remember that reality doesn't contain any concepts like "should" or "always." When stating reality, use only observable facts. It's much like presenting a case in court. It doesn't include any judgment about the circumstances. Judgments are the territory of the map. For example, if I were to state that a person said something hurtful to me, that wouldn't be an accurate statement of reality. Reality is only that a person said "X" to me. The "hurtful" part of the first statement is my map wanting to intervene.

2. After you have represented reality to the best of your ability, begin to write your judgments, feelings, and any mean-

ings you have about the event on a separate page. This is your opportunity to really vent. Include all the "shoulds" and "shouldn'ts." Include what the event means. Include why it is wrong, or why it is a problem. This is a representation of your map. It undoubtedly feels true to you. Remember that truth is defined by your map. Any adjustment to the map will feel at least slightly untrue in the beginning. Your gatekeeper hasn't allowed supporting information to enter.

3. Now, which are you able to change? Can you change reality? Can you change your map? Whichever changes, as soon as reality and your map are in agreement, the tension goes away. It's the rigidly held map that causes the most distress. A willingness to let go is needed in order for the map to rebuild itself in a way that can handle the situation. Ask yourself what part of the map would need to change in order to be at peace with the event. Peace doesn't necessarily mean that you like it or approve of it. Are you willing to entertain letting that part of your map go? Can you at least play with the concept?

Practice 15
MAPMAKING AT LEVEL 3

At level 3 it's not about pros and cons anymore. It isn't even about the map being in conflict with some outside event. It is an internal struggle. It's about higher and lower. Higher is closer to your ideal; lower is not. Lower may have seemed "right" according to your map, but now it's in question because you didn't personally create that portion of your map. This is where a personal value system begins to grow.

If you skipped over chapter 6, on intellectual intensity, it would help now to go back and read about values. Many of the internal struggles experienced at level 3 are about either the beginning of a change to the next value level or a mismatch between the value level of one's environment (family, work, church, etc.) and their personal value level. A value level contains not only values, but also associated beliefs, standards of behavior, and views of the world. Trying to hold your own personal value level while at the same time believing that you should "fit in" creates this level of conflict.

At this level it is necessary to find those deeper parts of the internal map of reality that no longer feel right. It's a time to discover and honor your personal values. While we retain the values from each value level as we progress, we also add new values. The important thing is to find the perspective that works. When moving from the blue to the orange value level, we don't have to abandon the important values from blue. Loyalty can still be important. But from the viewpoint of blue, the values in orange, such as independence and innovation, aren't given any importance. If you are moving into orange and trying to maintain a viewpoint of blue, you will be in extreme inner conflict. If you allow your viewpoint to move on to orange, the conflict can ease. That can be difficult if your surrounding environment is blue.

Another, and much more turbulent, entry into level 3 is when a traumatic event occurs. Any event that is life altering can force a jump to level 3. The death of a loved one or any other situation that causes one to question the meaning of life is a powerful force, made even more powerful by emotional intensity. Each time you've questioned your reason for living or the meaning of existence, you've been at the door of level 3.

This is the birthplace of existential angst. Existential angst has been described as the anxiety caused by the possible meaninglessness of existence. When we discover that all the meanings we have had throughout life are nothing more than an internal map of reality created for us when we were children, when those things we thought had meaning no longer do, when the emptiness is evident, how are we to feel but anxious? When meaninglessness collides with the pain of a sensitive person in an insensitive world, a true crisis is at hand. Many go in search of meaning, still hoping to find it "out there." To go on from this point requires a suicide of sorts. The old self must die, meaning that the old map must be allowed to fall apart. Remember that you are not the map. It is not you that is falling apart.

In Dabrowski's book *Existential Thoughts and Aphorisms*, written under the pseudonym of Paul Cienin, he said, "It is good that in society there are psychoneurotics and suicides. It speaks well for them—but not for the society."[32] His tenderness toward people at this step of emotional development reveals empathy born of his own internal struggle. Indeed, one looking at this moment in a person's life from the outside, completely removed from this level of angst, would label this a disorder, a mental illness beyond any question. But having been there, having gone through the abyss, Dabrowski recognized it in others and responded with compassion and wisdom developed through personal experience. He knew that it was a threshold to something greater, and at the same time he knew the intense suffering.

In a strange way, this point in time is liberating. The pressures that a person has endured due to the meanings society has put upon them are gone. The need to be a certain kind of person, possess material wealth, reach a certain level of success, or hold a position of importance evaporates. All meaning has been lost and, with it, all external pressure. The liberation is tempered, however, by the nothingness that remains. This is the night of the soul.

For a period of time, when you've let the old map go and you don't have a new element of the map to replace it, you will likely experience ambiguity.

1. Allow ambiguity: Tolerance for ambiguity helps. It can be built like a muscle with practice. The "practice" at level 3 is allowing ambiguity.

2. Trust that the map will resolve itself: The mind cannot tolerate ambiguity for too long, and before you know it there will be a new area of the map in place. In the meantime, an element of trust is required. Trust that the map will rebuild itself in that area, and trust that the new map will be better equipped to handle that situation and situations like it.

When you think about it, you've done this many times already. Whenever you encounter something new, something that takes you out of your comfort zone, you are dealing with ambiguity. Because the situation is new, you don't have an area for it in your internal map. With repeated exposure to the new situation, the map develops, making it more comfortable.

The dawn is the awakening of the authentic self. The meaning of life is being constructed again, this time at a higher level. Through self-education we explore with the fresh eyes of children. We find that there are higher things in life. We form ideals. Most important, we form a notion of an ideal self, a personality that incorporates the higher values, deeper awareness, and a richness of internal and external experience. This ideal is vague at first, ever refining, becoming more clear and concrete as time goes on. This is not removed from reality, but the seed of discovery of a higher level of reality. We have a new awareness of not only "what is" and "what will be," but also "what ought to be."

Practice 16
MAPMAKING AT LEVEL 4

In level 4 we begin a long road of adjusting ourselves to "what ought to be" and becoming maladjusted to "what is," or the common view of reality. We reject the lower parts of ourselves and of society in favor of the higher. The discernment of higher and lower is personal. This journey has no guide other than intuition. We demand more of ourselves. We strive toward perfection, only to realize how far we are falling from that goal.

At this level, the map takes on a different quality. It develops the same richness and depth on the internal as the map developed in level 2 for the external. There is "what is" internally, and there is "what ought to be." Instead of striving to recognize "what is" as the ultimate truth, we instead turn to "what ought to be" and work to bring about the change in ourselves. Parts of our old selves must die to make room for the new. We experience little deaths along the way, gaining trust that the death will bring new life with deeper meaning and higher moral values. The direction is no longer by chance, but focused with intention by our ideals. The map develops degrees of understanding of truth, beauty, and goodness. Just as the master cartographer is able to accurately represent a geographic area with creativity and aesthetic appeal, you too as a master mapmaker can represent reality in a creative manner that is appealing to your higher instincts and desire for fulfillment.

This level requires persistence and is punctuated with feelings of inferiority, both in relationships with others and with our ideal self-image. We continually deny and distance ourselves from lower instinctual behaviors in order to progress. When faced with a deep awareness of the ideals we value, we can't help but feel a sense of dissatisfaction with ourselves. An ideal, being so sublime, presents an unattainable goal, and as such, we can never hope to measure up. We must be willing to take stock from time to time and look at how far we have come. Measuring one's self against an ideal will always show a lack, a failure to have attained something. It will always appear to be as far away as it was at first conception. We can only measure our progress by looking backward, at the place we started. This should become a regular routine. We can become so focused and so dissatisfied with ourselves that we develop a habit of emotional self-flagellation. Declare a self-flagellation vacation! Rejoice in the progress along the path. Take stock of the depth of relationships formed. Celebrate the person you are becoming.

The practice at level 4 is to declare a breakdown. Since breakdowns are not happening to you spontaneously very often at this level, the road to growth involves creating a breakdown by declaration. If you search your inner experiences, you can usually find an area of life that isn't matching up to your ideal. Although breakdowns at this level are not the emotional roller-coasters they once were in levels 2 and 3, they can still be powerful. To declare a breakdown in that area involves only speaking it into existence. An example might be that your career isn't the one you would have chosen. It could be a case of "If I knew then what I know now, I would have done X instead. Now I'm too far down this path to change." By now you are getting much better at embracing a breakdown through the ambiguity and on to resolution even if that takes time. It is a matter of keeping the breakdown in mind, holding it carefully without forcing it to a premature solution.

A declaration is a speech act that has the power to create something. Declarations can always be followed by an exclamation mark. They have clarity and power. It may take time to formulate the declaration or it may come to you in a flash. Examples of declarations of this nature are "I refuse to do this anymore!" or

"My marriage isn't working!" or "I'm better than this job!" The key for the type of breakdown that pushes us further is to find an area of life that isn't in harmony with our ideal self. While it may be something that has been on the back burner, making the declaration about it brings it into focus. It pulls it from the back of the mind, the depths of the map, into consciousness. When the declaration has been made, we can look at the circumstances, the actions we've taken, or the judgments we've made and identify the area of the map that doesn't work with the image of our ideal self. There is an unspoken commitment by the ideal self that makes these circumstances, actions we have been taking, or meanings we previously held constitute a breakdown. What is that commitment?

At level 4 we make a conscious decision to give up the old identity, the old portion of the internal map, and the previous way of being, in favor of the new.

1. What commitment are you ready to make to move closer to your ideal self? Can you identify the possibilities that commitment would create? What actions are you prepared to take to honor that commitment?

2. Write down your breakdown declaration or work with a coach or mentor to whom you can speak these things. (Private, unspoken thoughts lack power.) The breakdown will show the area of conflict between your current self and your ideal self.

3. Articulate the commitment that would bring you in line with your ideal self.

4. Acknowledge the old part of your map that you are willing to erase. Be prepared for every part of your map that is not in agreement with your new commitment to stand up and be

counted. Ideas, beliefs, and parts of your self-image that you haven't examined in years, if ever, will show up to tell you why you can't make that commitment. These are the parts of yourself that you must be willing to let go. Mourn for them if you must.

4. List the possibilities that the new commitment would create for you. Be sure that you have clearly defined the commitment and that it truly is a part of your ideal self. The stronger the connection between the ideal self and the commitment, the more your emotions will support the commitment.

5. Finally, write the actions you are willing to take to honor that commitment.

Important Points for the Impatient

- Breakdowns occur as the internal map of reality is loosening. Each breakdown is actually an opportunity to adjust the map, resulting in emotional growth.

- Different kinds of breakdowns require different kinds of map adjustments. Each level of emotional growth is characterized by a different type of breakdown. The trick is identifying the type of breakdown and applying the corresponding practice.

- Level 2 breakdowns require an adjustment to the internal map of reality to better match reality.

- Level 3 breakdowns require the development of a more ideal self and a realistic look at how we may need to change to better match the ideal, a very personal part of the internal map of reality.

- Level 4 breakdowns are self-induced using a process called declaring a breakdown. These are intentionally created in order to further our growth.

15

The Ghosts of Intensity Past, Present, and Future

"Do you always have to have a purpose? Do you always have
to be so damn serious? Can't you ever do things without reason,
just like everybody else? You're so serious, so old. Everything's
important with you, everything's great, significant in some
way, every minute, even when you keep still. Can't you ever be
comfortable—and unimportant?"

"No."

—AYN RAND, *THE FOUNTAINHEAD*

There are many books that focus on how to overcome the challenges
of ADHD, but because it is viewed as a disorder, only the most
basic of challenges are addressed. So if you're interested in how to
handle the boring stuff of life without losing your mind, there are
already many wonderful sources for you. I'm more interested in providing information about the challenges that are not addressed by
people who consider intensity a disorder. Among the challenges I
hear about regularly are worry, being a perfectionist, and being too
serious. How many times has someone told you to "lighten up"? If
you're like me, it's become so familiar that you almost cringe at the

sound of it. Or maybe it's "Stop being such a perfectionist!" or "You worry too much!"

We do get tired of hearing these things from others. There are parts of each of these attributes that we hold dear. And there are parts of seriousness, perfectionism, and anxiety that present problems. Sometimes those problems are severe. I refer to these challenges as ghosts. They are invisible forces that influence us, sometimes consciously, but mostly unconsciously. The point of this chapter is to get to know each of these ghosts, these unseen forces that drive us, in a way that allows us to glean the best of them and exorcise the parts that don't serve us.

THE GHOST OF INTENSITY PAST: SERIOUSNESS

The ghost of intensity past is Seriousness. He's a favorite of mine. He gets things done and doesn't let anything or anyone get in his way. In many ways he's the poster child for intensity. He has found that by channeling intensity toward something, he can make better progress. He is the reason we sometimes intimidate others. He knows he holds that power. He also knows that he should be in charge and loves the feeling of working intensely toward something. He has a general disdain of triviality, preferring matters of importance.

The reason he is a ghost of the past is that he found a formula for success a long time ago, and we agreed. He has been with us for so long that we don't even notice his presence anymore. He brings seriousness as a winning formula to us daily now since it worked in the past. Our past experience with him and his success makes him a constant companion. His driven influence has been a part of our winning formula, the default methods and attitudes we use to succeed. He has been so invisible a companion, so much a part of our past, that we allow him into areas where he really isn't needed. Often we aren't even aware that he's taken over the wheel and is doing the driving.

Being serious, in and of itself, is not a problem, but being serious as a default creates the illusion that everything is important. This ghost of seriousness has trouble with degrees of seriousness. He takes it as either all or nothing. He can make being fifteen minutes late to a dentist appointment a grave event. The traffic on the road making you late can feel like the most important thing in the world at that moment. While logically we can differentiate between the seriousness of being late for a dentist appointment and missing a job interview when we've been out of work for months, he has trouble with the concept as evidenced by his actions.

The gift he brings is focus. His intensity is a powerful driver. If he is directed in areas of true importance, he displays a single-mindedness of purpose. He is passionate. If he is left to his own devices, he tends to spread his energy around, making anything in the current moment feel unduly important. When everything is important, it just becomes a way of being. It loses meaning. When he is given direction by the conscious mind on what is really important, he becomes a strong ally.

THE GHOST OF INTENSITY PRESENT: PERFECTIONISM

The ghost of intensity present is perfect, or at least she would like to be. She struggles over getting it right. She frets that it isn't good enough. While she spends a lot of time finding what's wrong with anything she's done, she sometimes produces excellent results. But she's never quite satisfied. It always could have been better. At times a task can seem so overwhelming to her that she just refuses to do it because she thinks she can't perform according to her own standards. She's big on ideals. Ideals are great because she can see such perfection in them. Never mind that ideals are unattainable. She's got a lot of energy and drive, and what's worth doing is worth doing with perfection.

You've got to love her. She's the one that made you stay up all night and get the term paper just right. Even though you got an A on it, she scolded that you could have done better. Still, the A is nice, and it wouldn't be there on your permanent record if she hadn't forced you to put all that time and energy into it.

She recognizes nothing but that which is or has the possibility of being perfect. In life, we get accustomed to thinking that nothing is perfect. However there is one thing that is now and will always remain perfect. That is an ideal. This is where the ghost of intensity present hides a gift for you. She understands and cultivates the possibility of an ideal. She believes it can be done. She has no concept of giving up.

Perfection doesn't come easily, or at all. But there is such a thing as mastery. To be an expert in one's chosen field provides the best chance to pursue perfection. In *Outliers*, Malcolm Gladwell shares that it takes ten thousand hours of practice to become an expert at something. That's eight hours a day, five days a week, taking off for a few holidays, for almost five years. In more realistic terms, if you were to work about twenty hours a week on developing some area of talent or expertise, allowing that you probably have a regular job taking up most of your time, it would take almost ten years to reach a level of mastery.[33] If this is even close to true, and he has some pretty convincing backing for the calculation, then we have to admit that we can't be masters of everything. There just aren't enough hours in the day.

The pursuit of an ideal is a noble endeavor, but the pursuit of every ideal means to squander the energy of the ghost. As I said, she has a lot of energy. She's not going to take a nap. If she has to, she'll pick at every trivial thing you do until you feel that you can't do anything right. She is strongest when focused in a single direction. Take the time and energy to focus her in a productive direction.

THE GHOST OF INTENSITY FUTURE: ANXIETY

This ghost is always worrying about the future. Unknown dangers and threats are ever present in his mind. He looks into the future and warns us of things that may happen. He spots potential threats everywhere. This ghost feeds off of intensity. The active intense mind and the active imagination support his need to imagine what may happen in the future. The sensual and emotional sensitivities provide him with experiences of pain to throw in our faces, proving his worth in his vigilant search for impending danger.

Once we've invited him in, he likes to stay. His story is that we can't get along without him, and he's pretty convincing. Every time we hear of any violence or misfortune befallen another, he tells us that it could have been us, if not for his efforts. Each incident that does affect us allows him to warn that we were not paying him enough heed. Whether we avoid a threat or a misfortune hits, he has a story about his worth. He tells how he either protected us or how he would have if we had only listened, and we believe him.

There are those who will say that anxiety is brought on by worrying. That is true sometimes, but just as true is that worrisome thoughts are generated when we're in a state of anxiety. One of the other causes of anxiety is excess psychomotor energy. Another cause is sensory overload. Anxiety is a common attribute of intense people. In fact it is the primary reason that we are able to develop further than others. Anxiety helps to bring on breakdowns, which are a loosening of the internal map of reality. It actually assists in bringing a breakdown to the point of growth. With sufficient anxiety over a breakdown, the internal map of reality falls apart, and a new part of the map is able to create itself.

Anxiety also creates another potential gift for us. Within anxiety is the intense desire to take action. When anxious feelings are too general to recognize a specific threat, that need to take action is stifled because there is no clear action to take. However, when we can see a clear danger, anxiety fuels our ability to jump into action. When we move into action toward a worthwhile endeavor, anxiety turns to exhilaration.

As you can see, anxiety is not the devil we once assumed. He's a more benevolent ghost than one would imagine. He is always ready to protect you and warn of potential threats. He drives you to growth, even when you go reluctantly, and he fills you with energy when there is something that can be done to bypass danger. It's just that when he's not being fully employed toward some goal, he finds his own way of keeping busy. This is when he fills your mind with imagined problems, eats away at your stomach, and sometimes makes you ill.

HOW TO BE THE LEADER OF THE GHOSTS

The three have much in common. They are all born of intensity. They are all persistent, defying attempts to be subdued. They are all able to either make us extremely successful or cripple us, depending on our willingness and ability to be in the lead.

They can't be allowed to run amok. When they are moving together toward a worthwhile endeavor, they are the best of allies. When they are free to wander and entertain themselves, they can be troublesome. If we can create more balanced relationships with each of them, we can benefit from the gifts they provide and avoid the pitfalls. The trick to building more balanced relationships is to be in the driver's seat. We need to give them focus. Each of them does extremely well for us if, and only if, they are working on our agenda. They are not to be banished but to be better understood and invited to work with us.

These ghosts must be led with finesse. They have already proven that they aren't easily managed. As long as you approach them with a command-and-control style of management, they will rebel. You can count on it. They must be led the same way people are led. Give them a vision of a future they can all be excited to be a part of, and call on them to use the strengths only they can bring.

The ghost of perfection is the first in the lineup. When you have crafted the ideal vision, she is the one who will hold it. She will use all her powers to keep the ideal foremost in your mind and compare the steps you're taking against it. She'll let you know when you've gone off the path.

Next, the ghost of seriousness will keep this vision as important. He can stop making every little thing important, because he finally has a mission. It gives him the perspective he needed all along, and he will be most grateful for it. Once he has his place in realizing the vision, he brings passion to the lineup. While his considerable power to drive toward a purpose is focused on the vision you've provided, you will receive the relief that can only be felt when he gives up the little things. I'm sure you've heard the saying that there are only two rules in life: "Don't sweat the small stuff," and "It's all small stuff." Almost true. There is only one thing that doesn't fall into the category of small stuff. You get to decide what that is. Seriousness will support you all the way.

Finally, the ghost of anxiety will be called upon for two things. He must continue to alert you to areas for growth. Every time you run into a stumbling block to moving forward with your vision, he must provide the incentive to grow past it. He has an uncanny ability to recognize when something is right or wrong and speak to you with a gut feeling. At the same time he will provide the energy to take action. He can use his incredible muscle to build a feeling of unease to propel you forward whenever you aren't moving in a positive direction toward the vision you created.

Important Points for the Impatient

- Seriousness, perfectionism, and anxiety are all attributes of intensity that are sometimes sources of suffering and at other times assets depending upon our relationship with them.

- Taking the lead in these traits allows one to reduce or entirely eliminate the negative effects and put them to work in creating whatever we decide we want in life.

16

Living an Intense Life

Here's to the crazy ones, the misfits, the rebels, the troublemak-
ers, the round pegs in the square holes, the ones who see things
differently. They're not fond of rules and they have no respect
for the status quo. You can quote them, disagree with them,
glorify or vilify them. About the only thing you can't do is
ignore them, because they change things. They push the human
race forward. While some may see them as the crazy ones, we
see genius. Because the people who are crazy enough to think
they can change the world, are the ones who do.
—APPLE COMPUTER INC. AND STEVE JOBS (1955–2011)

Intensity doesn't go away. It's not a temporary condition from which
to be cured, nor is it a stage to be outgrown. It is as much a part of
you as body, mind, or heart. Whether you live that intensity as a
curse or a blessing is up to you.

These things we've experienced—the wounding caused by care-
lessness, by people unaware of how easily we bruise, the burning
passions that drive us to joy and just as easily to near insanity, and
the separation of being so different (the separation is perhaps the
worst), these and more—make us who we are. We are complex. We
are fragile, and strong, challenged sometimes by simple tasks and
creative geniuses all at the same time. We walk on tiptoes, afraid of
being noticed, and then stomp with such determination the world

shakes. Intensity, which is the seed from which we grew, continues to form who we are becoming.

Some have soared, spreading wings and flying above all the labels and nonsense. No diagnosis stops them; no institution cages them. They charge forward, being sure somehow that the uniqueness of their being is inherently worthy. Others have cowered, aware only of the pain of being different. The tentative steps their spirits have taken out into the world have been quickly retracted as soon as the first blow of insensitivity is dealt. They live quietly inside, pretending, always pretending to be like the others. The difference between one path and the other is determined by three things: understanding your intense nature, having a source of support, and taking action.

UNDERSTAND YOUR NATURE

Without a deep understanding and acceptance of your intense nature, you can easily be convinced that you have a disorder. With it, you can step out into the world, perhaps for the first time, unapologetically authentic.

If we were not a minority of the population, these things would be common knowledge. Schools would teach according to the type of learning we do naturally. Emotional development would be as common in our continuing education as history or math. The environment would be created in a much more sensitive fashion in order to preserve a sense of safety and comfort. But this is not the case. Because we are such a minority, and because we haven't been aware of each other, we believe our differences to be inadequacy. We experience these differences as very personal, thinking that we are alone in these intensities.

Each time you've read a refrain and thought "How did she get inside my head" or "I thought that was just me," it is another kernel of proof that you are not alone. In fact, you are in very good company. If you can find accurate biographies of people who have brought significant change into the world, you'll see proof of intensity throughout their journeys.

This book is a step along the way to understanding and accepting your true nature. Understanding how your body works as the unconscious mind and how your gatekeeper forms your experience of the outside world is the beginning. Through this understanding you can begin to take proper care of yourself. Having a more accurate model of how your mind works allows you to capitalize on your strengths of nonlinear thought and creativity. The important step of self-acceptance is dependent upon having a frame of reference for powerful moods and emotions that provides both the understanding of why you are the way you are and a path of development introducing some level of control over the emotions you entertain while leaving intensity intact.

This first component of understanding your nature can make the difference between a self-image of disorder and a new self-image of uniquely gifted. This is not a small thing. At this point many people are able to go back and reevaluate memories of their lives starting with childhood according to this new deeper understanding. That's when it becomes very clear that they were never disordered or broken. They have always been sensitive and intense, and the events of life up to this point were experienced without that knowledge. Up until this understanding is felt in the bones, life has been lived as though we should feel, behave, and think differently than what is normal for us. We've been pretending on some level and, through that pretending, denying our true nature. This is when we get to stop.

FIND SUPPORT FROM OTHERS

No matter how much you understand yourself, intensity continues to be intense. Feelings can still overwhelm. Being intense is not easy.

The kind of life where there is no questioning, no anxiety, and little to no turmoil is not in the cards for us. We need a soft place to land. We need someone to pick us up when we've fallen and sometimes to encourage us on. We need support.

Support comes from people, only from people. They can be others who understand and value your intensity. They can be friends or family who may not always understand you but always love you and are willing to support you as you continue to grow. Or support can come from therapists or coaches, provided they have an understanding of intensity as something other than disorder. Dabrowski believed that the most effective path for intense people to grow and develop was what he called "self-therapy." He understood that he, as a therapist, didn't have all the answers for all the people. He knew that each person would have to find their own way. He also knew that they needed support as they went through this. This combination of reframing what would have previously been considered psychoneurosis into more accurate and understandable terms of "super-stimulatability"—or "intensity" in my terms—and support was the most effective way to help his gifted and creative patients.

For therapists and coaches I recommend reading as much as you can find by Dabrowski himself. There is something about his writing that imparts the compassion he felt for the people he treated. He himself was intense and had personally been through emotional, creative, and intellectual development. Traditional therapy and coaching is less suitable for intense people, as it can serve to reinforce feelings of inadequacy. If you find that some of your patients or clients are intense, they may be best served as Dabrowski's patients were, with reframing and support.

Support can also be found in books like this book, right here and now. You'll find that a lot of intense people write books. They don't have to be self-help books. Any book by or about an intense person can provide a level of comfort and support. This need for support doesn't leave us when we reach some magic age or level of development. This is for a lifetime. Because of that, it makes sense to find those sources of support now and nurture them.

TAKE ACTION

People come into their own at different points in life. For the intense person it's a little later. For example, a "normal" person may choose a direction in life, complete an education in support of that direction, and be fully engaged in their field of choice by their late twenties. The amount of focus and direction they display seems incredible to many of us. Then by the time we are in our forties or fifties, we've found the same kind of focus and direction. Why does it take us longer? We simply have more complex equipment, and it takes more practice to master it. Think of it as driving a race car as opposed to driving a regular car. With just a little practice, people are able to master the type of physical and mental coordination required to drive a normal car. To drive a race car requires additional training and a lot more practice. Our bodies, minds, and emotions are more like a race car. They go faster and they are much more complex.

The timeframe for the intense person to reach a level of mastery over their own equipment can be shortened. I think that if we were in the majority, the practices needed to learn to use our intense minds, bodies, and emotions would be considered basic education. Since we are in the minority, we are left to our own devices. That normally means that we have to gain the experience by trial and error through living. The practices that have been presented here are designed to speed the process.

The third and last thing that makes the difference between soaring and cowering is taking action, both to engage in the practices that cause you to grow and further develop and to plan and take action toward some goal, ideal, or direction in life. Only you can make the decision to take action. This is the point where you decide your future.

For some, it may seem too late to finally finish an education, embark on a new career direction, or pursue some purpose in life. It may seem that there is a specific time in which that sort of activity is allowed and that time has passed. I can tell you that if you are still breathing, you still have time. An intense person of any age who is able to hold a single ideal in mind and take action toward that ideal will have a profound impact. This is fact.

CONCLUSION

Through the new understanding you have of intensity, you now have a different way of looking at yourself, at your family, and at life's possibilities.

It's time to stop viewing yourself as disordered. There is no need to measure yourself according to standards designed for a different type of person. If you were diagnosed with ADHD or another mental disorder (in reality a warped and incomplete view of intensity), it may have come as a relief at first. It meant that you were not to blame for not fitting in. It meant that you couldn't help it, and that someone else, a doctor or therapist, was responsible to fix you or at least explain your limitations. Now that you understand the real underlying condition, the responsibility is back on you. You are no more to blame for the way you are different than you were when you thought you were disordered. The biggest difference is being able to see the whole picture, the gifts associated with intensity as well as the differences that cause discomfort. It means that you are back in control of your life with tools to create the life you desire, free from labels of disorder.

EPILOGUE

I hope that you have found a better understanding of yourself and come to realize why I value you so much. My intention is to enable you to see yourself in a new light. You are indeed a special kind of person whose gifts have from time to time been called "disorder." Each of the intensities brings something special to you. They provide power and sensitivity. They are the reason for your undeniable creativity, your passion, and the complexity of your character. It has been my privilege and pleasure to share this journey with you.

ACKNOWLEDGMENTS

To my sister, Karen Masinter, for providing support both in editing and spirit. I love you.

To my love, Carl, who put up with me being overextended for a year without complaint.

To my friend Carol Courcy, who made me believe in my own possibilities.

And a special thank-you to my son Adam for telling me the brutal truth about the content. You have him to thank if you have not been bored while reading this.

NOTES

1. "A.D.D.—A DUBIOUS DIAGNOSIS?" The Merrow Report, *PBS NewsHour*, PBS, aired October 20, 1995, transcript, Attention Deficit Disorder, *www.add-adhd.org/ritalin_CHADD_A.D.D.html*.

2. *www.chadd.org*.

3. Rachael Rettner, "Steady rise in use of ADHD meds in kids, teens." *My Health News Daily*, MSNBC.com, September 28, 2011, *www.msnbc.msn.com/id/44699488/ns/health-childrens_health/t/steady-rise-use-adhd-meds-kids-teens/#*

4. Dr. Joseph L. Humpherys, MD, "Stimulant Medications Increase Risk for Sudden Death in Children," February 14, 2011, Ezine Articles, *ezinearticles.com/?Stimulant-Medications-Increase-Risk-for-Sudden-Death-in-Children&id=5864972*.

5. American Psychiatric Association, "Homosexuality and Sexual Orientation Disturbance: Proposed Change in DSM-II, 6th Printing, page 44," position statement, APA Document Reference No. 730008, 2.

6. Allen Frances, "It's not too late to save 'normal,'" *Los Angeles Times*, March 1, 2010, *articles.latimes.com/2010/mar/01/opinion/la-oe-frances1-2010mar01*.

7. S. N. Visser, MS, et al, "Increasing Prevalence of Parent-Reported Attention-Deficit/Hyperactivity Disorder Among Children—United States, 2003 and 2007," Centers for Disease Control

and Prevention, *Morbidity and Mortality Weekly Report* 59 (44), November 12, 2010, 1439–43.

8. National Institutes of Mental Health, statistics page, accessed February 2011, *www.nimh.nih.gov/statistics/index.shtml*.

9. Gretchen B. LeFever, Andrea P. Arcona, and David O. Antonuccio, "ADHD among American Schoolchildren: Evidence of Overdiagnosis and Overuse of Medication," *The Scientific Review of Mental Health Practice* 2 (1), Spring/Summer 2003, *www.srmhp.org/0201/adhd.html*.

10. Sami Timimi, *Child Psychiatry and the Medicalization of Childhood* (Hove, UK: Brunner-Routledge, 2002).

11. Susan Daniels, PhD, and Michael M. Piechowski, PhD, eds., *Living with Intensity: Understanding the Sensitivity, Excitability, and Emotional Development of Gifted Children, Adolescents, and Adults* (Scottsdale: Great Potential Press, Inc., 2009).

12. Candace Pert, *Molecules of Emotion: Why You Feel the Way You Feel* (New York: Scribner, 1997).

13. C. E. Kerr et al, "Effects of mindfulness meditation training on anticipatory alpha modulation in primary somatosensory cortex," *Brain Research Bulletin* 85 (3–4) 2011, 96–103.

14. Jeremy Gray, "Meditation Associated with Increased Grey Matter in the Brain," *Yale News*, November 10, 2005, *news.yale.edu/2005/11/10/meditation-associated-increased-grey-matter-brain*.

15. National Center for Complementary and Alternative Medicine, "Meditation: An Introduction," National Institutes of Health, NCCAM pub no. D308, last modified June 2010, *nccam.nih.gov/health/meditation/overview.htm*.

16. Massachusetts General Hospital, "Mindfulness meditation training changes brain structure in eight weeks," *ScienceDaily*, January 21, 2011, *www.sciencedaily.com/releases/2011/01/110121144007.htm*.

17. Mark Wheeler, "How to build a bigger brain: Study shows that meditation may increase gray matter," *UCLA Newsroom*, May 12, 2009, *newsroom.ucla.edu/portal/ucla/how-to-build-a-bigger-brain-91273.aspx*.

18. Guiseppe Pagnoni and Milos Cekic, "Age effects on gray matter volume and attentional performance in Zen meditation," *Neurobiology of Aging* 28 (10) October 2007, 1623–27, *www.science direct.com/science/article/pii/S0197458007002436*.

19. Elaine Aron, *The Highly Sensitive Person: How to Thrive When the World Overwhelms You* (New York: Three Rivers Press, 1998).

20. Jerome Kagan, et al, "Temperament and Allergic Symptoms," *Psychosomatic Medicine* 53, 1991, 332–40, *www.psychosomatic medicine.org/content/53/3/332.full.pdf*.

21. Alan Fischman, MD, et al, "Dopamine transporter density in patients with attention deficit hyperactivity disorder," *The Lancet* 354 (9196), 1999, 2132–33, *www.sciencedirect.com/science/article/pii/S0140673699040301*.

22. Aron, *The Highly Sensitive Person*.

23. *Dictionary.com*, s.v. "urge," accessed October 24, 2011, *dictionary.reference.com/browse/urge*.

24. NIH/National Institute of Mental Health, "Cortex Matures Faster in Youth with Highest IQ," March 29, 2006, *www.nimh.nih.gov/science-news/2006/cortex-matures-faster-in-youth-with-highest-iq.shtml*.

25. Pat McCaffrey, "Little Einsteins: High IQ Linked to Plasticity in Young," Schizophrenia Research Forum, March 31, 2006, *www.schizophreniaforum.org/new/detail.asp?id=1255*.

26. Bruce D. Perry, "Traumatized Children: How Childhood Trauma Influences Brain Development," *The Journal of the California Alliance for the Mentally Ill* 11 (1), 2000, 48–51.

27. J. Madeleine Nash, "Fertile Minds," *Time*, February 3, 1997, 49–56.

28. Willem Kuipers, *Enjoying the Gift of Being Uncommon: Extra Intelligent, Intense, and Effective* (Voorberg, Netherlands: Kuipers & Van Kempen, 2010).

29. Don Edward Beck and Christopher C. Cowen, *Spiral Dynamics: Mastering Values, Leadership, and Change* (Oxford: Blackwell Pub, 1996).

30. Harry Nilsson, script, *The Point*, directed by Fred Wolf (1971).

31. W. Tillier, "The basic concepts of Dabrowski's Theory of Positive Disintegration," unpublished manuscript, "Perspectives on the self: Proceedings of the Second Biennial Conference on Dabrowski's Theory of Positive Disintegration," Alberta, Canada, June 22–26, 1996.

32. Paul Cienin, *Existential Thoughts and Aphorisms* (London: Gryf Publications, 1972) 34.

33. Malcolm Gladwell, *Outliers: The Story of Success* (New York: Little, Brown and Company, 2009).

ABOUT THE AUTHOR

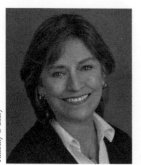

Martha Burge is an ADHD coach, mother to two sons diagnosed with ADHD, and a very intense person. She holds a BA in Psychology, an MA in Organizational Development, and is certified as a personal and professional coach by the Newfield Network. She writes on the subject of ADHD for examiner.com and has spoken to local chapters of Children and Adults with ADHD (CHADD) on the moods and emotions of ADHD. She is active in the Mensa community and is a trusted ADHD coach to Mensa members.

After raising two very intense sons and working with coaching clients, she found that by raising awareness of the underlying condition of intensity, she was able to help people who previously thought of themselves as broken find a new self-image. The success of this approach was too good to limit it to her coaching clients. She had to write this book.

Martha Burge lives in Southern California. You can visit her at *www.intensitycoaching.com.*

TO OUR READERS

Conari Press, an imprint of Red Wheel/Weiser, publishes books on topics ranging from spirituality, personal growth, and relationships to women's issues, parenting, and social issues. Our mission is to publish quality books that will make a difference in people's lives—how we feel about ourselves and how we relate to one another. We value integrity, compassion, and receptivity, both in the books we publish and in the way we do business.

Our readers are our most important resource, and we appreciate your input, suggestions, and ideas about what you would like to see published.

Visit our website *www.redwheelweiser.com* where you can learn about our upcoming books and free downloads, and be sure to go to *www.redwheelweiser.com/newsletter/* to sign up for newsletters and exclusive offers.

You can also contact us at *info@redwheelweiser.com.*

Conari Press
an imprint of Red Wheel/Weiser, LLC
665 Third Street, Suite 400
San Francisco, CA 94107